21 DAY KETO DIET AND INTERMITTENT FASTING FOR RAPID WEIGHT LOSS

KETOGENIC DIET PLAN: GET IN THE ZONE TO DETOX, RESET AND CLEANSE YOUR BODY, BURN FAT AND MAINTAIN YOUR GOAL WEIGHT

LISA SCOTT

TABLE OF CONTENTS

INTRODUCTION

Everyone wants to lose weight, but not everyone wants to go through the challenges that the process of weight loss entails.

It's one thing to put your body through the struggles of strenuous exercise, but following a restrictive diet can be challenging for the best of us.

Unfortunately for those trying to achieve a full body transformation, the diet aspect of weight loss efforts make up 75% of results.

In fact, countless individuals have managed to trim down their waistline, and achieve a full body transformation, just by making a few changes in the kitchen.

But everyone knows it's not that easy. According to surveys, dieting is often considered more difficult than exercise, because it pushes people to sacrifice something they enjoy.

Food, aside from being a biological need, is something that we tend to associate with festivities, fun, friends, and family.

It's not surprising then, that when we to cut down on food intake, avoid certain types of food, and follow a strict eating schedule, it can make what was once an enjoyable part of life, feel like a chore or even dreary.

In an attempt to make dieting more appealing to those of us who need to lose weight, doctors and diet experts have pitched in to give their opinions.

Their efforts have birthed literally hundreds of different diet strategies over the years. No matter how enticing and easy they're made to seem, one thing's for sure - results are never guaranteed.

The problem with fad diets is that most of them were developed without sound nutritional guidance and theory.

For instance, the low-fat diet, a popular strategy often said to be effective at quick and easy weight loss, might sound like a sound weight loss solution. But is it really?

When confronted with the word "fat," people think overweight, obese, or in extreme cases, even ugly. So any food that contains "fat" should be avoided in order to reduce weight and achieve a slimmer, more appealing appearance. But science would tell you otherwise.

Eating a diet that lacks enough fat obligates people to consume more carbohydrates. When broken down, these carbs are turned into glucose which travels through your bloodstream and triggers the release of insulin. This hormone ferries blood glucose to the tissues and organs where it's needed.

When a person consumes an excess of carbohydrates, the extra sugars are stored as fat for later use which makes the entire concept of a low-fat diet counterintuitive.Worse still, a high-carb diet can cause cravings.

Packing lots of carbs over a single meal can cause a sudden rise in blood glucose. Once the sugar concentration in your blood falls, you're likely to crave more carbs, eat more than you need, and feed into the vicious cycle of fat storage.

Ironically, over time, a low-fat diet can actually cause you to gain more weight than you started with, defeating the purpose of a diet altogether. Unfortunately for a lot of those who bought into the low-fat diet craze, this information wasn't widely available when it was first conceptualized.

But now, research into the way our bodies work has revealed the flaws of the low-fat diet. And what has surprised both experts and laypeople is that the exact *opposite* of a low-fat diet is actually what works best for weight loss - the high-fat diet.

A major game-changer in the world of weight loss comes in the form of the ketogenic diet.

It was initially developed in the 1920's and 30's, knowledge on the keto diet was largely kept hush-hush, because it wasn't really intended for mainstream use. But after it was featured on *Dateline* and in the made-for-TV movie, *First Do No Harm*, the strategy started gaining popularity until it became a full-blown weight loss trend that shows no signs of abating.

INTRODUCTION

As the complete opposite of the low-fat diet, the keto diet works by encouraging dieters to eat a larger proportion of fat in their meals, compared to both proteins and carbs.

For many, this seemed like a surprising way to lose weight, but thousands of real-life keto diet success stories are testimony to the success of this approach.

The appeal of the keto diet mainly stems from the fact that it doesn't impose unrealistic calorie restrictions, it doesn't keep people from eating the food that they enjoy, and it doesn't require strict meal schedules.

The keto diet lets dieters enjoy food, without having to feel guilty about the food they eat or the amount they consume.

So in a sense, it's reimagined the way we see diets and made it possible for people to lose weight without being unhappy in the process.

Put simply, the keto diet has managed to sustain its mainstream prominence, simply because it works. Thousands have achieved quick and easy transformation through adopting the keto diet.

And maybe that's why you're here.

Perhaps you've been disappointed by diet plans that have come and gone without results. Maybe you're tired of feeling unhappy about what you see in the mirror? Maybe you just want to do what's best for your body.

Whatever your reason, the ketogenic diet might be just the answer you're looking for.

If you're fed up with putting all your effort into a weight loss plan that doesn't deliver, maybe it's time to try something new.

In this comprehensive guide, you'll learn everything you need to know about the ketogenic diet. You'll discover how it started, why it works, and how you can apply it in your life, to achieve the benefits that it promises.

So, if you're ready to turn those dreams for transformation into tangible realities, let's get started.

INTRODUCTION

1

WHAT IS THE KETOGENIC DIET?

The ketogenic diet is a high-fat diet that encourages the body to produce ketones.

Initially, the keto diet was developed for individuals with epilepsy and similar seizure disorders. In the 1920's and 30's, the ketogenic diet was used as one of the cornerstones of the treatment of epilepsy in children. According to research, these molecules have the potential to manage seizures with their powerful anticonvulsant effects.

Today, the ketogenic diet has made a comeback as one of the most popular diet trends of the modern age.

Since hitting the mainstream market, the keto diet has seen unprecedented popularity. It's front and center, as one of the most effective weight loss strategies we've seen in the last 30 years.

While being an effective diet should be reason enough for its popularity, there are a few other things about the keto diet that make it stand out in a sea of hyped-up weight loss strategies.

Keto Promotes Eating more Fat

Not long ago, people would have probably laughed at you if you told them you were on a high-fat diet. But now, that's what almost all weight loss hopefuls are putting into action.

The fact that the keto diet doesn't tell you to eat less fat makes it controversial - a factor that has led to the development of its cult following.

We're conditions to think that more fat in your diet should make us more fat, but something about the way the keto diet works produces the opposite results.

With such an uncommon mechanism, the diet strategy piqued the interest of hundreds of thousands of dieters, blasting it off towards worldwide popularity.

Keto doesn't Impose Impossible Restrictions

Consider the Paleo diet - another fad diet that came and went in the early 2000's. Developed in the 1970s, this weight loss strategy required its followers to avoid any food that our cavemen ancestors from the Paleolithic era might not have consumed.

Essentially, you would have to assume what early cavemen might not have had access to, and what specific food choices they had.

So aside from the food itself, certain meal preparation methods would also be prohibited under the strict rules of the Paleo diet. On top of that, conventional cooking essentials like cooking oil would have to be replaced with the caveman equivalent. Certain spices and condiments might also be defined as unacceptable.

But because most of our food comes from grocery stores and supermarkets, it becomes difficult to curtail every single item in your cart to make sure you're following through the way you should. Plus, there's a lot of the decisions you'd make would have to rely on your own assumptions. Did they have kosher sea salt back in the paleolithic era? Unless you brushed up on your studies of prehistoric man, questions like that might be hard to answer.

On the other hand, most diets revolve around restricting calorie intake, restrictive meal schedules, and food choices so drastic or boring, that eating ends up feeling like a chore.

Conventional diets often have high expectations of the dieter. After all, it's often our lack of self control that's meant we're overweight in the first place! Expecting us to exercise self-control for a prolonged period of time is simply unrealistic.

It's these expectations of self-control, and following a detailed plan, that is ultimately what pushes us off the wagon, causing us to give up before we see any real weight loss results.

The beauty of the keto diet is that it doesn't curtail food choices the same way other fad diets do.

It lets you eat good food, continue to enjoy celebrations, and make daily meal prep choices that don't require all of your time and energy.

Ingredients are easy to source, recipes are practical and do-able, and the food itself resembles what you would typically eat.

Keto Satisfies your Hunger

Most dieters will agree that they can call a day a success if they were able to battle their cravings and suppress their appetites.

That's what most diets will do to you - impose strict limitations that starve you and have you feeling hungry for long periods throughout the day. That's hardly sustainable for any of us, no matter how strong our willpower.

Many diets work by widening the deficit between how much you consume and how much you burn, as the way towards effective weight loss. The reality is that those of us who need to lose weight, just don't have what it takes to control hunger.

If you're relying solely on your diet for weight loss, then it becomes harder to create a larger deficit, since you're not performing any exercise to burn more of the excess.

Suppressing hunger pangs is more than just mind over matter. Hunger can continue to take a toll on your mood, mindset, and disposition as you proceed to ignore it. If you're sensitive to your sugar levels, you may even feel confused or angry, and unable to make decisions well.

We owe this to our body's negative feedback mechanisms - the more you withhold a response, the more it heightens the stimulation, in an effort to receive a response. In this case, the stimulation is hunger, and the response is whether or not you choose to satisfy it with food.

Perhaps the biggest selling point for the keto diet is that it doesn't tell you how much you can eat.

In fact, many keto experts and guides will tell you that the keto diet lets you eat as much as you want. Despite this, overeating becomes an unlikely mistake with this specific weight loss strategy - whether or not you watch out for the possibility.

It's all in the way that the keto diet works, satiating your hunger and keeping you feeling full for longer compared to most diet plans.

Comparing the keto diet to all of the other popular diets that have earned similar popularity, it's hard not to see how it changes our perception of how diets should be. This non-restrictive strategy makes it easier to maintain the diet throughout the process of weight loss.

Ultimately, this is made possible by the fact that the keto diet doesn't aim to produce a deficit between what you eat and what you burn - or at least, not directly. So the amount of calories you consume isn't the focal point of the process.

So how else can a person lose weight if not by reducing the amount of calories they eat?

The keto diet's physiological mechanism can answer that question.

How the Ketogenic Diet works

On the surface, there are a few things about the ketogenic diet that are generally known to most of those who've heard of it - whether or not they've actually tried the method themselves.

For instance, the ketogenic diet:

- doesn't focus on caloric intake or metabolism

- encourages more fat consumption

- satisfies hunger and keeps you feeling full for longer

- works for most body types

These snippets aren't new. In fact, most of those who try to sell the idea of the keto diet will weigh down on these points to get their message across.

While it's all good and well to know what the ketogenic diet does, it's doubly important to know how the keto diet does it.

Sure, not everyone can be a physiology expert, and certainly not everyone wants to be. But, understanding how the diet works will make it easier to pattern choices throughout the process, in order to support this weight loss strategy's unique physiological mechanism.

The Problem with Your Normal Diet

The best way to truly understand how the keto diet works is to first figure out how the body operates, and how conventional dietary choices that we make when we're not on a diet can affect it.

Visit any elementary school classroom, and you're likely to find the iconic Food Pyramid. It's the same food pyramid that's been used for years, even though scientific research has shown that much of what's included to be outdated.

The Food Pyramid was designed to help give us a clear cut idea of what food we need to eat and how much of each food group our bodies require.

This chart puts 'Go foods' as the base and foundation of any healthy diet. In essence, 'Go foods' are carbohydrates - starchy, sugary, fiber-rich foods that provide us with the energy we need to accomplish different bodily functions.

These 'Go foods' come in a wide variety and are typically taken with other foods to give people the feeling of being full. From pastas to rice, white bread, grains, and cereals, carbohydrate-rich foods give us sugars which are used as energy on a molecular level.

According to most of those who abide by the guidelines set forth by the traditional Food Pyramid, the Go foods should make up the largest portion of a person's diet, amounting to 65-75% of their typical meals.

While there isn't anything inherently wrong with the intake of carbohydrates, it's worth mentioning that eating too much can be problematic.

When we eat carbohydrates, they're broken down in our digestive system and turned into sugars - particularly, glucose. This is then transported into our blood where it's collected by insulin to be ferried off into different tissues and organs. Once at their destination, sugars are used as molecular energy, allowing a variety of bodily functions to occur.

If we eat too many carbohydrates, insulin takes the sugars in our blood and stores them away as fat for future use. This is our body's programmed mechanism, centered on reducing waste and preparing for any potential future deficits.

While a little stored fat should be no problem, consider what would happen if an individual were to consume an excess of carbohydrates every day. Those needed by the body would be used, but those that exceeded the requirement would be stored away as fat.

As days pass, the storage centers become satiated with sugars tucked away as lipids or fats, which ultimately lead to weight gain.

Unless you're doing something to burn away what's been stored, your body will just continue to accumulate fat throughout the different storage centers distributed throughout your system.

The problem with eating a diet that's mainly composed of carbohydrates, is that it doesn't put any emphasis on the maintenance of a healthy physique. Of course, it supplies you with the energy and sustenance you need now, but if you eat too much of it, you end up gaining weight. And unfortunately for those who observe this standard diet, overeating is a real possibility.

Studies have found that a diet rich in carbohydrates puts a person at risk of a sugar crash. Hours after a high-carb meal, an individual's blood glucose can crash dramatically, leading to hunger cravings, and a sudden appetite boom.

In many cases, the body signals for the intake of even more carbohydrates, in order to raise the levels of blood glucose, which is why individuals might crave specifically for carb-rich choices. And so the vicious cycle continues.

Anyone trying to lose weight and maintain a slim, fit physique can see how a high-carb diet can be an unforgiving downward spiral into continued weight gain. But from the perspective of health, there are other dangers that come hand in hand with an excessively carb-heavy diet.

Global statistics published by the World Health Organization revealed that the incidence of diabetes has risen from 108 million in the 1980's to 422 million in 2014.

These numbers continue to soar, with the occurrence of diabetes across the globe exponentially increasing. Of course, there are numerous factors that could result in the development of diabetes. But, as the years continue to roll on and our dietary practices change, it seems that becoming diabetic is more and more likely.

Aside from being a precarious diet for those who want to stay slim, a carb-rich diet also puts people at risk of developing chronic hyperglycemia. Increased blood sugar levels over a long period of time can damage the blood vessels and cause problems in the function and production of insulin.

Once this happens, an impairment in blood glucose management can lead to full blown type 2 diabetes - which is the 7th most deadly disease worldwide.

As if that's not reason enough to avoid the factors that might lead to diabetes, it's also worth mentioning that it's also the most expensive disease to manage, costing sufferers $327 billion USD annually in the USA alone.

Does this mean that you need to cut carbs completely? Not at all. In many cases, the food you eat will always contain, to some extent, some amount of carbs. These can be used as a viable energy source and work great for those times when you might need a quick energy fix. But as a lifelong dietary staple, carbohydrates can be dangerous in the long run.

While it's clear, a diet that demands a person eat 65-75% carbohydrates daily, can be a weight watcher's nightmare, the question remains - why should you focus on eating more fat?

If the goal of weight loss is to burn existing fat storage and prevent fat from being stored away, then why would a fat-rich diet be the right solution?

The answer might surprise you.

The Keto Diet Mechanism

The keto diet attracted quite a bit of attention when it was first popularized as a mainstream weight loss diet, because of its unconventional requirements.

Calling for more fat, than both carbs and proteins combined, the mechanism that the diet employed towards weight loss was a massive mystery to most of those who wanted to lose an extra tire.

But there's a lot of sound evidence and scientific truth to the way that the keto diet works, making it a suitable weight-reduction strategy for those who want to lose weight fast.

The first principle that explains the efficacy of the keto diet is the fact that fat - when consumed - doesn't turn into sugars when metabolized. Eating mostly fat decreases the amount of glucose in our bloodstream. Without an excess of glucose, insulin won't have anything to store.

On top of that, a lack of glucose prompts the body to look for energy elsewhere. And that's where the fat reserves come into play.

The body puts excess glucose into storage in the form of fat, so that the body has a supply of energy at the ready in case of emergencies. These include instances when there might not be enough carbohydrate intake, so the body metabolizes fat stores and turns them into ketone bodies. These ketones are used as energy molecules, forcing our bodies to run on a process called ketosis.

The process might happen to you regularly when you miss a meal or two, but what the keto diet does is force the body into a continuous state of ketosis.

Essentially, the strategy starves the body of carbohydrates over an extended period of time, forcing it to burn fat, in order to fuel the different processes it needs to accomplish. Despite that, the keto diet keeps you feeling full and satisfied, since high-fat foods typically take longer to digest, compared to carbohydrates.

Now, here's the big question you're probably wondering about - should you cut carbohydrates out of your diet completely?

While the ketogenic diet imposes very high portions of fat per meal, it doesn't wipe out carbs entirely. This is because the brain runs better on carbs because they're faster to burn and process, and readily changed into glucose. Since the brain requires lots of energy at a fast pace, carbs make the better energy source. So the keto diet does allow the consumption of at least some carbs to provide the needs of the brain.

Benefits of the Keto Diet

Obviously, the main objective of those who take on the ketogenic diet is to lose weight.

With hundreds of thousands of others who have successfully achieved the physical transformation they'd long hoped for with the help of keto, there are millions more who are in pursuit of the same results.

Of course, there's more to it than just anecdotal evidence - but the numbers don't lie. Studies conducted in 2013[1] proved that very low carbohydrate ketogenic diets were much more effective at weight loss than their low-fat diet counterparts. In the clinical setting, ketogenic diets have also been used to counter obesity and diabetes.

Based on scientific evidence collected through a number of studies, the ketogenic diet works best to reduce weight, when observed diligently over a short period of time. The process of ketosis is effective as a quick weight loss fix, but also poses a few dangers, if prolonged (more details on this later).

Although the reason of weight loss might be good enough to give the ketogenic diet a try, it actually offers a few other advantages that make it a suitable wellness strategy as well.

Heart Health

Some studies[2] have found that the ketogenic diet shows a few unique benefits for those who might be at risk of cardiovascular disease.

The fact that it can help reduce weight in obese individuals already makes it a viable solution against the complications of heart conditions. But more than that, it also directly improves the health and function of the heart.

Long-term studies that observed the effects of a ketogenic diet on participants, over the span of 3 years, revealed improved cardiac risk factors. The diet can lower triglycerides, normalize blood pressure, and improve glycemic management. This is mainly thanks to the fact that fat can come in the form of high-density lipoproteins (HDL).

Foods like avocado, olive oil, legumes, nuts, and salmon are some of the main food choices that people observing a keto diet can indulge in. These foods are rich in HDL - otherwise called the good cholesterol.

Working to sweep through the bloodstream and remove bad cholesterol (i.e. VLDL, LDL), HDL prevents the accumulation of atherosclerotic plaque - a pathological collection of cholesterol that risks vascular disease and cardiac arrest.

Of course, not all fatty foods are packed with HDLs. While most of the fat-rich food choices available will provide the same ketogenic effects, and thus weight loss, not all of them present the same advantages for heart health.

Choosing the right fat-rich foods and avoiding those that contain too much low-density lipoproteins will help make the method more beneficial for cardiovascular health.

Liver Health

The liver is one of the organs in the body that's most prone to excessive fat storage. As the main processing center for all the different food that you eat, the liver makes the ideal storage center as well, since anything and everything you consume will pass through it.

If your body detects that the food you've eaten exceeds what your system needs, it holds it as fat in the liver, where it will be kept for future use.

Glucose and low-density lipoproteins are the molecules that typically make up the fat stores in our liver. As these accumulate, individuals run the risk of developing fatty liver disease - a condition characterized by an overly fat-padded liver with impaired functioning. Untreated, fatty liver disease can be fatal.

While there are a number of available treatment options for individuals suffering from the condition, it's been found that fatty liver disease might actually be effectively addressed by a high-fat diet. Foods rich in high-density lipoproteins can clean away the accumulated fat from the liver, and restore its functioning to normal levels.

One study[3] conducted on individuals with fatty liver disease aimed to see the benefits of a ketogenic diet on the condition. After observing the diet for 6 months along with supplementation, the participants showed significant histologic improvements verified by post-treatment liver biopsies. Moreover, the respondents also achieved dramatic weight loss results, which helped improve their overall health and wellness, to support the positive effects of the diet on their livers.

Cancer

Global reports estimate a whopping 20 thousand daily deaths as the result of different kinds of cancer, placing the annual death count at around 7.6 million. Also worthy of note, the World Health Organization estimates 12 million new cancer diagnoses in the coming year. While these numbers are quite staggering, there are studies that suggest that 30-40% of cancer deaths can be prevented, and that 30% of all cancer diagnoses can be significantly tempered, and even cured, with timely treatment.

In March of 2017, over 80 new generation cancer medications were approved for medical use. These drugs aim to help manage the condition and fight back the growth and proliferation of new cancer cells. Unfortunately, while some of these new pharmaceuticals might be promising, their efficacy ultimately depends on how well a person's system will take to them.

Some studies have found that new generation cancer medications might only be able to provide marginal positive changes, which seem counterintuitive given their dramatic list of side effects and adverse reactions.

In light of this, researchers have tried to find new ways to make cancer medications more effective and, as their studies would prove, the ketogenic diet might be a suitable adjuvant therapy for cancer treatment.

According to studies, cancer cells might owe their growth and propagation to the presence of glucose. Much like all the other healthy, normal cells and tissues throughout our bodies, cancer cells need sustenance to feed off of and survive.

Of course, that source has to be an energy-giving molecule that's available in large quantities, to be able to sustain growth. Glucose is a widely bioavailable energy source throughout our bodies, and cancer cells have found them to be ideal for growth.

In fact, research has found that cancer cells uptake glucose 10-15 times more aggressively than healthy, normal cells in our bodies. This can be proven with PET scans - a test that requires patients to ingest radioactively labeled glucose, which gets preferentially absorbed by cancer cells, making it light up on a scanner.

Given this information, it can be said that removing glucose from a person's diet can starve cancer cells of the energy they use to grow and spread. Of course, this doesn't eliminate the cancer altogether, since some research has found that cancer cells can also use other energy sources, such as amino acids for growth. However, decreasing glucose intake does help decrease the rate of cancer growth.

On top of that, it has also been found that cancer cells prefer acidic environments. Unfortunately for high-carb dieters, sugars come with an acidic pH balance of 6.4 - ten times more acidic than the ideal blood pH balance.

In large concentrations, high glucose levels can cause a systemic acidic blood pH balance - one of the cornerstones of an ideal environment for cancer growth. In terms of the immune response, sugar has also been found to cause unwanted and possibly dangerous effects.

Our bodies naturally enact phagocytosis - a "Pac-man" process that eats away unhealthy, damaged, and irreparable cells. In some cases, an increased intake of sugar could reduce phagocytosis by up to 50%.

Phagocytosis is important because it cleans away any unnecessary cells. Because cancer cells start out as defective cellular growths, phagocytosis becomes a necessary process to kill them off and clear them away, before they accumulate and form a tumor.

Unfortunately, individuals with high blood glucose might not be able to reap the optimal benefits of phagocytosis, decreasing their capacity to address early cancer growth by 38-50%.

One study aimed to find the connection between a sugary diet, cancer growth and prognosis. The systematic review[4] took into account information from several other studies to determine a correlation between cancer growth and a carb-rich diet.

Based on the data collected, it was discovered that a ketogenic diet can dramatically lengthen survival rate and decrease the rate of tumor growth in a variety of cancers.

Some studies also found that a keto diet could help improve the efficacy of several cancer drugs, allowing them to provide more potent, significant effects.

Skin Health

As an individual continues to load carbs into their diet, they enter a state called pathological hyperglycemia. Characterized by high levels of blood glucose over a long period of time, this state can cause damage to the different factors that play a role in the process of glucose metabolism.

Once the body reaches its breaking point, it develops insulin resistance which simply means that the body is no longer able to use insulin as it normally would. This leaves more glucose in the blood, which can damage vital organs and other tissues throughout a person's system.

Aside from causing problems with glucose regulation, insulin resistance also rears its ugly head in other ways. A study published in 2015[5] was able to determine the role that insulin resistance plays in the development of severe acne.

The relationship can be attributed to the fact that insulin can signal the production of a variety of other hormones in the body. When a person's system becomes resistant to insulin, the body might call for an increased production to make up for the inefficient functioning. This increases levels for other hormones, causing an outbreak of acne.

Other than that, high-density lipoproteins (which are found in fatty foods) have also been found to work wonders for the skin. These molecules improve overall skin health and appearance, and even help with wound healing.

So bumping up the fat in your diet and cutting back on sugary carbohydrates can help prevent or reverse severe acne, and help make skin more radiant and clear.

Mood Normalization

On a high-carb diet, it's very possible to experience dramatic mood changes throughout the day.

This is the result of the rising and falling of blood glucose as you eat, burn, and store sugars from the carbohydrates that you consume.

During episodes of hyperglycemia (that is, high sugar levels), you might notice difficulty concentrating, fatigue, and headaches, while episodes of hypoglycemia (that is, low sugar levels) might have you feeling irritable and anxious.

Normalizing your blood sugar should help eliminate the effects it can cause on your mood. By indulging in a diet that's mostly made up of fats, your body has a more stable energy source, preventing the effects associated with the dipping and spiking of glucose in your blood.

Some studies[6] have gone as far as discovering the connections between a high-carb diet and depressive symptoms. The correlation stems from the fact that foods that rank high on the glycemic index, tend to fuel the production of chemicals and hormones that have been linked to depression.

What's more, the unstable nature of glucose puts individuals prone to unstable emotions as well. One minute, their brain functions are aptly sustained, and the next, they're starving for more carbohydrates.

While experts on the ketogenic diet admit that carbohydrates are a good source of energy for brain functions because they're easy to burn, metabolize, and use, a diet that depends solely on carbs for energy can cause dramatic mood swings, more often than preferred.

Getting accustomed to a fat-rich diet can help make for more stable cognitive and emotional functions.

Weight Loss

Above any other benefit that the keto diet might provide, it's most widely appreciated for its capability to reduce weight over a short period of time.

Sure, many of us hope to achieve weight loss for the aesthetic benefits, but there's a lot more to a normal body weight than just an improved appearance.

Excess weight and obesity are the second leading cause of a variety of preventable diseases - these include cardiovascular conditions, diabetes, and stroke.

Too much stored fat interferes with normal bodily functioning, impairing a variety of biological processes and leading to severe outcomes and repercussions later on.

What's nice about the ketogenic diet is that it lets you lose a significant amount of weight in just a short period of time.

For those who need the benefits of fast, safe weight loss, the diet proves to be a reasonable strategy.

As with any diet, it's not without its dangers. But when correctly and appropriately used, the keto diet can be a major game-changer for your health and wellness.

1 https://www.cambridge.org/core/journals/british-journal-of-nutrition/article/verylowcarbohydrate-ketogenic-diet-v-lowfat-diet-for-longterm-weight-loss-a-metaanalysis-of-randomised-controlled-trials/6FD9F975BAFF1D46F84C8BA9CE860783

2 https://www.ncbi.nlm.nih.gov/pmc/articles/PMC5452247/

3 https://link.springer.com/article/10.1007/s10620-006-9433-5

4 https://www.ncbi.nlm.nih.gov/pmc/articles/PMC5450454/

5 https://www.ncbi.nlm.nih.gov/pmc/articles/PMC4565837/

6 https://www.ncbi.nlm.nih.gov/pmc/articles/PMC2738337/

LISA SCOTT

2

CHOOSING THE RIGHT
KETO DIET FOOD

The keto diet's popularity stems from the fact that it essentially asks people to eat *more fat* - something that most individuals initially thought they had to avoid in an effort to lose weight.

Although it is true, in essence, that the keto diet calls for more fat, when you're eating for ketosis, there are only certain types of fatty foods that you should include.

What is Good Fat?

Good fat - also called good cholesterol - is high-density lipoprotein (also known as HDL). These HDLs are found in certain types of fatty foods, and provide us substantial benefits across the board in terms of our health.

What's particularly beneficial about HDLs is that they take away bad cholesterol. Essentially, HDL works by moving through your system, collecting bad cholesterol, and sweeping them out to take them back to the liver.

This prevents cholesterol from building up in your blood vessels - an issue which can lead to cardiovascular disease later on.

On a keto diet, you should be focused on eating food that contains good cholesterol in order to reap the benefits that the diet promises.

Sure, you may still lose weight even if you indulge in bad cholesterol (or LDL), but the effects that the diet can have on your health may be dramatically reduced. In extreme cases, an LDL-rich keto diet might even cause you harm.

What is Bad Fat?

Low-density lipoproteins (known as LDL's) are the opposite of HDLs, and they cause significant danger to our health and wellness over time. It's this type of fat that accumulates in our blood vessels, causing the formation of atherosclerotic plaque.

If, and when, this build-up of fat dislodges from the vessels, it can travel through the bloodstream, cause a blockage, and kill off tissues of certain organs. When it blocks a vessel that supplies the heart, you suffer what's called a myocardial infarction: a heart attack. When the vessel blocked is responsible for providing blood to parts of the brain, you suffer a stroke.

Again, eating a diet that's mainly composed of bad cholesterol can still provide you with the weight loss effects you're looking for. But because of the dangers that this type of food can pose when it comes to your health, it's suggested that you avoid them altogether or at least try to minimize your intake.

Tips on Choosing the Right Keto Food

There's a lot more to choosing keto-friendly food aside from just checking the labels.

Sure, there's a lot to learn from taking a closer look at what the packaging has to say.

But you're are urged to avoid taking nutritional information at face value, since they might require a bit of interpretation. For instance, typical store-bought almonds might indicate a carbohydrate content of around 9 grams per 100-gram serving. Most Keto dieters would see this bit of information and quickly put the item back on the shelf, because it exceeds the ideal amount.

However it pays to look into the fiber content before actually making a decision. As a general rule, not all of the carbs listed in a food item will be absorbed into your system. The fiber portion will simply pass through your digestive tract, so it won't be taken up as glucose or stored as fat.

So to get a more accurate carbohydrate content, subtract the fiber content from the total carbs to arrive at the net carbohydrate content.

With the above example, you might find a fiber content of around 5 grams with your typical store-bought almonds, placing the net carbohydrate content at just 4 grams per 100-gram serving.

Now, doesn't that seem like a suitable pick for your keto pantry?

What Foods are Best for keto Diet?

The bane of most dieters is the lack of food choices for certain weight loss disciplines. With such a bland selection for daily menus, dieting might seem like an absolute chore.

But that's where the keto diet takes the proverbial cake once again, providing dieters with a wide selection of food items that can be combined, cooked, and prepared in a multitude of ways, to give you a menu that's ever changing, fun, and of course, enjoyable.

Fish and Seafood

One food item that keto dieters can really enjoy, and come up with a variety of tasty dishes, is seafood.

Most types of fish are packed with micronutrients, and have virtually zero carbohydrates. Some choices - like salmon, trout, sardines, and tuna - are also rich in good cholesterol (or HDL's), which is why they've become staples for keto dieters.

In the seafood department, there are also a variety of choices that suit the keto diet parameters. Shrimp contains virtually no carbohydrates, while choices like squid contain as little as 3 grams of carbs for every 100 grams. Then there are some with a higher carbohydrate content, such as mussels, which contain up to 7 grams of carbs per 100 grams.

Keep in mind that while most types of fish and seafood are made up mostly of HDL's, there are some that contain other components as well, like proteins and carbs.

If you're trying to adhere to a very low carbohydrate keto diet, then it may be important to consider how these numbers can add up, if taken with other foods that contain small amounts of carbs.

Low-Carb Vegetables

Vegetables are common ground among different dietary strategies.

Made up mostly of fiber and micronutrients, vegetables don't really contain a lot of fat per se, but they do fill up the gap when it comes to your need for vitamins, minerals and micronutrients

Some of the best vegetables to include in a keto diet include:

- cauliflower

- broccoli

- zucchini

- celery

- spinach

- cabbage *and*

- asparagus

Of course, even these vegetables contain some carbohydrates, ranging from 2.9 grams to 3.5 grams per 100-gram serving. However, they provide necessary fiber and micronutrients that you, as a keto dieter need and won't easily be able to get elsewhere.

Low-Carb Fruits

Fruits are probably the keto diet's bulwark, simply because of the fact that this is the food group where you might find one of the most powerful ingredients in any ketogenic meal - the   avocado.

Rich in HDL, the humble avocado is a fat-packed fruit that can be prepared and enjoyed in a variety of ways.

Aside from the avocado, there are some other fruits that you might want to include in your meal prep plans.

Choices like olives, berries, and citrus fruits are wonderfully flavorful ingredients that you can use to bump up the flavor of the meals you make for your keto journey.

Eggs

There are a multitude of ways that eggs can be prepared, making them one of the most versatile foods included in the list of ideal choices for the keto diet.

Each egg contains less than 1 gram of carbohydrates for every serving, and is made up mostly of fat and protein.

Typically, dieters are encouraged to steer clear of fried eggs because while it does meet the macronutrient parameters for the ketogenic diet, they might not be as healthy as other methods of preparation.

As a general rule, poaching is the most ideal process of preparation, followed by hard-boiled, and then scrambled.

Cheese

There's a wide variety of cheese, and several of them prove to be great choices for those who want to adhere to the keto diet.

Cheddar, brie, goat, blue, parmesan, and mozzarella are some of the fattiest types of cheeses, with as little as 0.1 gram of carbs per 100-gram serving. These ingredients add a punch of taste to an otherwise bland meal and make typical keto meals more exciting and enjoyable.

Of course, it's worth mentioning that cheese is known to contain quite a bit of sodium, as well as bad types of fat, depending on the specific type.

That said, adding it into your diet as a flavor booster, rather than as a staple ingredient, can make help balance out the negative effects it might have on your health.

Greek Yogurt

Whether as a dressing, a sauce, or a snack all on its own, Greek yogurt is a staple food choice in any keto dieter's refrigerator. Sure, it's not really rich in fat, and it might have quite a few carbs in there. But it's protein content makes it a viable ingredient for more than a few ketogenic recipes.

For every 150 grams of plain Greek yogurt, you get about 5 grams of carbs and 11 grams of protein.

Aside from its ideal macronutrient profile, Greek yogurt also helps suppress your appetite and keep you feeling satiated and satisfied for much longer.

Olive Oil

Another way that you can adapt to the ketogenic diet would be to observe keto-friendly meal prep choices.

So, instead of just using any regular cooking oil for your recipes, consider choosing olive oil which is rich in monounsaturated fats.

In fact, olive oil has been proven to be made purely of fat, so it fits the ketogenic diet perfectly. Extra virgin olive oil is a variation that also meets ketogenic standards, while adding a few other benefits.

For instance, the extra virgin formulations are high in antioxidants - compounds that help provide a number of health benefits throughout the different systems in your body.

Nuts and Seeds

Making a great snack for those on a keto diet, nuts and seeds comprise a large number of recipes that you might find circulating the web.

Upon doing a little research though, you might have found that some nuts contain up to 12 grams of carbs per serving - like chia seeds.

So, how do they manage to wiggle their way into very low carb ketogenic diets? The answer lies in the fact that they also contain high levels of fiber.

So in the example of chia seeds which contain a whopping 12 total grams of carbohydrates for every 28 gram serving, only 1 gram actually remains in your system. The rest of the 11 grams of carbohydrates are fibers which won't be absorbed by your body.

So, nuts make a great addition to your ketogenic recipes. Adding a few walnuts, almonds, pecans, or chia seeds to your meals can make for interesting textures and flavors, and can assist in promoting healthy bowel movements.

Unsweetened Chocolate

So what about those with a sore case of sweet teeth? Should chocolate treats be scratched out of the grocery list forever?

Fortunately for chocolate lovers, there are ketogenic alternatives that can still give you that daily dose of chocolatey goodness, minus the guilt of carbs.

Unsweetened chocolate contains just 3 grams of carbohydrates for every ounce (or 28 grams), so it really works well as a chocolate flavoring for keto treats and goodies that you might want to concoct in your kitchen.

Of course, you need to think of the workaround for the sweetness factor though, since unsweetened chocolate might not be too palatable on its own. Nonetheless, there are keto-friendly sweeteners, which can be mixed into your recipes to give you authentic baked goodies minus the guilt.

Meat and Poultry

The keto diet isn't all fat. Remember, a portion of your diet will be dedicated to protein, so it's important that you get some meat and protein in there.

For every 5 grams of meat, you get zero net carbs, which makes it a great addition to your meals especially if you're looking for something extra filling or savory.

Keep in mind though that when you choose your meat, you should try to find grass-fed options instead of grain-fed. These meats have much more omega-3 in them and provide better health benefits for those on keto.

It's also worth mentioning that the way you cook your meat plays a role in the nutritional value it brings to the table. For instance, breaded meats and poultry recipes can add a significant amount of carbohydrates to your meals.

Another thing to consider is how frying can increase the fat content in your food, which might seem like a good option for those on keto.

However, because the oils that are most viable for the ketogenic diet have low smoke points, there might be some technical skill required to fry foods using these oils.

What Foods to Avoid?

Just as you would probably want to stock up on the choices listed above, there are a few grocery store items you might want to say sayonara (or goodbye) to, once and for all.

These food choices can work against your keto diet efforts no matter how healthy and viable they might seem as ketogenic choices.

Starchy Vegetables

If you're adding vegetables to your keto diet, it's worth noting that there are still some choices that you might want to steer clear of.

These include starchy vegetables that pack carbohydrates in large quantities. As you might have already guessed, some examples include potatoes, yams, corn, yucca, parsnips, and beans.

One serving of a potato-laden dish can have you soaring way beyond your ketogenic boundaries in just one sitting.

So as a rule of thumb, if it grows in the ground (with the exception of corn), it would be in your best interest to seek other choices.

Dark Chocolate

If unsweetened chocolate makes a good choice for keto, then dark chocolate shouldn't be too far behind!

Of course, taste and texture wise, there's not too much of a difference. So how different can they be nutrition-wise? Before you start short-cutting your way through those baked recipes you've found through your favorite keto gurus, consider the fact that dark chocolate goes through a completely different process.

Even dark chocolate choices that use up to 80% pure cocoa for their formulation, can contain as much as 10 grams of carbohydrates per 28 grams. So, before you switch out the unsweetened for the dark variation, in the hope of cutting back on stevia, then you might want to consider the carbohydrate discrepancy.

Watermelon

Mainly made up of, well, water, surely the watermelon makes a great ketogenic ingredient or snack?

Unfortunately, while it does shine with the qualities of what you might expect a good of a good keto choice, watermelon actually contains around 8 grams of carbohydrates for every 100-gram serving.

It's not really up there compared to starchy vegetables, sure. But if you consider that there are a lot of other fruits out there that provide the same refreshing taste, minus the high carb count, then watermelon becomes an obvious no-no for die-hard ketogenic dieters.

Sliced and Shredded Cheese

Ah yes, cheese - the friendly flavor-adding ingredient that every keto dieter should have in their fridge.

While we all love our daily dose of delicious cheese, you might want to make sure you're getting it as natural as possible.

Cheese that's not processed and that adheres to the traditional preparation methods are best for keto dieters because they don't include any other ingredients that could be detrimental to keto.

For instance, shredded cheese - those that can be purchased in packs in the grocery store - actually contain quite a bit of potato starch to give flavor and texture. The result? A large carbohydrate content that defeats the purpose of the low-carb concept.

Soy Milk

Made from beans, low-carb, and possibly organic? Soy milk sounds like the *perfect* addition to your keto diet, doesn't it?

Before you go stocking up on soy milk on your next grocery trip, consider this - there are healthier options out there.

While it isn't recommended to stay on a ketogenic diet for prolonged periods of time, choosing the healthiest foods during your diet will help prevent a lot of the health complications that a carb-rich diet would cause.

Unfortunately, soy milk can be highly processed, which highlights the presence and effects of stomach irritants and hormones which could even mess with a woman's menstrual cycle.

In this light, it's also worth mentioning that other foods made of soy should also be taken out of your diet, such as tofu, soybean oil, and soy-enriched protein powders.

Wine

Fermented grapes? Surely, wine should be a ketogenic food! While no one wants you to have to give up your weekly wine fix, there's some pretty bad news you need to be aware of - most wines aren't actually keto friendly.

But you did the research - wine contains only 2.7 grams of carbohydrates for every 100-gram serving. How could it not be a keto-friendly choice?

The answer lies in the fact that during the metabolism of alcohol, you end up with by-products that could interfere with normal biochemical pathways. That's why you end up feeling a little tipsy or disoriented after a few drinks.

Your body's main function then shifts from burning lipids, glucose, and amino acids, towards burning the by-products of alcohol consumption.

So what happens? All the other macronutrients are put on hold and possibly stored in order to burn away the molecules generated from alcohol metabolism. This puts a dent in your body's learned metabolic speed (which you worked hard for with your ketogenic diet efforts), and slows down fat-burning over a long period of time.

Depending on how much alcohol you've consumed, you might have to wait a whole day before the process normalizes and your body returns to its usual metabolic rate.

Cashews

Everyone knows that nuts are some of the best foods to snack on if you're on a keto diet. Made up mostly of fat, the carbs in nuts can be easily factored out if you consider the presence of fiber, which isn't actually digested or absorbed into our system.

So despite the pretty steep total calorie count, cashews should be a safe zone for keto dieters. Right?

Wrong! Unfortunately, cashews have very little fiber, if any. So that total carb count you see is actually pretty close to the actual net count. For every ounce of cashews, you get a total of 10 carbs before subtracting fiber, and a net of 9 carbs after.

Now, because those numbers can add up pretty quickly, chomping down on even just a few cups of cashews in a day can have you way beyond your carb limit in no time.

Legumes

Beans are one of the main staple foods that vegans and vegetarians include in their diets because they're versatile, and they can be prepared to mimic a variety of meats and other animal products.

While they are healthy in general, they do pack quite a large amount of carbohydrates per serving. For instance, the humble chickpea - the main ingredient in hummus - contains 61 grams of carbs for every 100-gram serving.

Avoiding them in your keto diet should help keep you within the carbohydrate limit.

Grapes

Sweet, small, and juicy, most would think that grapes make an ideal ketogenic snack. But at 17 grams of carbohydrates for every 100 grams, it doesn't really make such a great choice if you're looking for something that will satisfy very low carbohydrate parameters.

A better alternative would be blackberries, which contain as little as 6 grams of net carbs after factoring out their fiber content.

And the list goes on

Of course, this list isn't all inclusive, and some of the choices might find a place in your diet as long as you know how to manage your macros. So how can you make sure?

The best way to guarantee that you've got a grocery cart, full of keto-friendly food is to do your research.

There are a lot of food choices out there that don't provide enough information on their labels, so lots of buyers are left standing in the grocery store aisles wondering whether or not to toss it in their cart.

Everything - from those big staples like bread and rice, down to the little added flavorings like seasonings, sauce, and spices - can all contain carbohydrates. Even if they're in small amounts, grams

LISA SCOTT

can add up and push you over your boundaries, making it very possible to get kicked out of ketosis, even if you were trying to be careful.

This is one of the reasons why dieters are urged to plan their meals ahead. Researching your choices and figuring out what you intend to prepare for the upcoming weeks can make it a whole lot easier for you to avoid any food that doesn't fit the parameters of keto.

This also keeps you from tossing non-keto friendly food in your shopping cart, thinking that it would have fit your diet even if it actually doesn't.

Remember, keeping an eye on your carbs is tantamount to weight loss in the keto game.

So it's essential that you take extra care when making the right grocery store choices. With that, it's probably only appropriate to discuss just how that can be done by managing your macros.

Managing Your Macros

Macronutrients are basically large energy molecules that fuel the different biological functions that your body performs. These are different from micronutrients, which essentially help promote proper cellular health.

Perhaps one of the hardest things to master, when it comes to starting your ketogenic diet, is understanding how macros work.

For a keto diet to be considered successful and authentic, an individual must follow a specific division of macronutrients, in order to achieve the benefits that the diet promises.

Generally, the breakdown of macros on a typical keto diet entails 65-80% fat, 15-30% protein, and 5-10% carbohydrates. This percentage pertains to the amount of calories you have in a day.

According to experts, quantifying the amount of each macronutrient in the form of grams can be tricky since everyone is different.

But as a baseline, most individuals are encouraged to consume a maximum of only 50 grams worth of total carbs (or 20-30 net carbs) in a day.

For protein, the measurement can be slightly easier to figure out. Experts recommend only around 1 gram of protein per kilogram of body weight per day. So if you weigh 60 kilos, you can consume around 60 grams of protein each day.

Whatever is left of your caloric intake, after subtracting the grams of protein and carbs, should be made up of fat.

Maintaining these numbers can help keep your body in a state of *ketosis* during which it burns more fat, as it looks for an alternate energy source due to the lack of carbohydrates. In some cases, an individual might be able to maintain ketosis, even if they take in as much as 80 grams of carbohydrates.

It really varies from person to person, so you need to fully understand your metabolic rate, your caloric intake, and your body's response to the diet, before coming up with foolproof numbers for your macro-management.

As a general rule, individuals who tend to gain weight more slowly, are better adapted to eat slightly more grams of carbohydrates, even if they're on keto.

To figure out if you're one of them, consider this checklist:

- You've only gained around 20 pounds over the span of 2 or more years
- You're known to eat a lot, yet maintain a slim figure

- You exercise intensely regularly and incorporate weight lifting into your workouts

- You have a stable, routine sleeping schedule that rarely or never gets interrupted

- Your base metabolic rate is relatively high

Individuals who store fat less readily are more capable of burning up carbs faster, so they don't risk falling out of ketosis, even if they eat around 30 grams of extra carbohydrates in a day.

3

HOW TO FIRE UP YOUR METABOLISM

The ketogenic diet, on its own, can be a suitable weight loss strategy, and has been proven as one through research and scientific study.

In most cases, the ketogenic diet has been used as a weight loss tool for obese individuals, who might not be able to lose weight with traditional means like exercise.

Although it is quite an effective method without the need for ancillary efforts and practices, the benefits of keto become much more pronounced when you toss in a few exercise strategies that bump up your metabolic rate.

These tactics make it possible to fire up ketosis to burn more fat stores and lose more weight over a short period of time.

Cardio Exercise

When we engage in high intensity, demanding exercises like weight lifting, our bodies rely on glycolysis to generate the energy needed to sustain the exercise.

It isn't until after around 2 minutes of effortful exercise that our bodies will tap into fat reserves. So, if you were to weight lift without enough carbs in your system, there wouldn't be a resource for glycolysis.

Thus, you would struggle to achieve optimal performance, and perhaps even injure yourself along the way without burning any fat stores.

That said, experts recommend that individuals undertaking a ketogenic diet observe cardio workouts instead. Low-intensity jogging, swimming, or cycling, for instance, can be much less demanding on your body.

This means they can be sustained for longer periods, keeping you moving and active beyond the two minute time-frame it would take to tap into fat reserves. Engaging in 30-minute cardio sessions each day can significantly bump up your rate of weight loss by 30-40%, depending on how often you exercise.

You can also try scheduling your workouts earlier in the day so that you can burn more calories as you go about your usual activities.

For those who can eat more carbs or protein without interfering with ketosis, it might be possible to engage in high intensity interval training. Quick bursts of higher intensity between low intensity cardio can help you burn even more.

Just make sure to keep the bursts to a maximum of 15 seconds, to keep yourself from feeling too tired too soon.

Supplements

There are some supplements in the market that are said to boost metabolism in a variety of ways, depending on how they're formulated.

One of the more popular ways that supplements aim to speed up a person's metabolic rate is by increasing body temperature.

It's a little complicated as to how this actually works, but experts say that it has something to do with the amount of kinetic energy that's available to cells.

Your body regulates everything that happens to your system, including your body temperature. By increasing the heat, your body works harder to keep everything at equilibrium, allowing you to burn a little extra, even during idle moments.

Does it make a monumental difference? Not really. But the minor shift can bring about significant change, when added to other metabolic adjustments you make.

Move Around

Experts have dubbed sitting as the new smoking, saying that it's one of the unhealthiest habits of the modern day.

A sedentary lifestyle, that keeps you seated or motionless for long periods of time, can slow down your metabolism. This is because a lack of physical activity simply means a lack of the necessity to burn calories, since there's nothing that needs to be fueled other than your involuntary bodily functions.

Standing up and moving around your space at regular intervals can help significantly increase your metabolic rate.

Engaging in short bursts of aerobic exercise can make a great solution to end a sedentary session. Every 30 minutes, consider standing from your desk and walking around your office space. You can take a flight of stairs up or down from your floor, and return to your workstation afterwards.

If you've got a more private space, you might want to consider stretching and limbering up, to give your muscles a break from the lack of movement.

Sleep on Schedule

Researchers have found a link between lack of sleep and obesity.

In some studies, poor sleeping habits have also shown a connection to insulin deficiency and increased blood glucose levels.

When a person doesn't get enough sleep, they experience an increase in the hormone ghrelin which causes the feeling of hunger. In the same light, they also tend to go through the day with decreased levels of leptin, the hormone responsible for giving the feeling of fullness after a meal.

Experts recommend that adults sleep for at least 8 hours straight every night. This helps normalize metabolism and control eating habits for the day ahead.

Many studies have exposed that proper sleeping routines can actually help a person burn more calories at a regular pace, since their body was given a well-deserved tune-up the night before.

Eat What You Need

One of the most basic principles that dieters tend to observe is eating less. Not wanting to load more calories than are burnt, even some keto dieters fall for this often damaging dietary technique.

The thing about starving your body of calories - regardless of what form they come in - is that it takes a toll on your metabolic rate. If your body detects that you're not receiving enough fuel to fire up the different biological processes it needs to get done, it will cut back on calorie burning.

This is its natural survival strategy which it enacts to make sure you have enough energy to see you through the day, under the assumption that you won't be getting any more any time soon.

When deciding how many calories you should be consuming in a day, remember that there is no magic number. In fact, with the keto diet, knowing your caloric intake has less to do with setting a limit, and more to do with understanding how to divide your macros.

If you know how many calories you need, you can more properly assign your fats, proteins, and carbs. Counting calories for the sake of restriction isn't actually recommended on keto, for one reason - eating mostly fat will help you regulate more easily, because it's easier to feel full after a meal.

People on keto rarely ever eat more than they should, since fat satiates hunger more effectively than any other macro.

If you need to know the most appropriate caloric intake for your specific needs, you can find a calorie calculator on the web.

LISA SCOTT

These take your weight, age, height, gender, and level of activity into account to give you an estimate of the proper number of calories you need in a day. Some calculators might also provide you calorie counts for losing weight and gaining weight.

4

THE KETO EFFECT - WHAT TO EXPECT AFTER 21 DAYS

So, you've successfully managed to stay on track for 3 weeks.

By this time, you might be noticing a few changes in terms of how your body looks and feels.

In fact, some of those who have gone on keto claim to have seen changes as soon as 7 days after dedicating themselves to the diet. While it is different for everyone, it's uncommon for differences to take more than a month to show, especially if you've been doing it right.

Now, what exactly can you expect out of your efforts closing in on the 3-week mark?

Increased Energy Levels

At the start, you might feel your energy sputtering and your body being slightly more sluggish than usual. But, as the days roll on and you stay dedicated to your new diet, you might begin to experience higher levels of energy to see you through your usual schedule.

Experts attribute this to your body becoming accustomed to its new main energy source. Generally speaking, fat can be much more stable than glucose as a source of energy, because it doesn't dip and spike like sugar does. Fat reserves are available throughout your body, and will always be at the ready when needed. This is opposed to glucose, which only becomes available when you eat.

With a much more stable energy source providing a reliable stream of macronutrients to your system, you'll start to feel more energized, since your body should stop experiencing sugar crashes and spikes brought about by glucose intake.

Loss of Appetite

Perhaps one of the most pronounced changes that a keto dieter might experience, after 3 weeks of staying on track, will be a decreased appetite.

When you stuff your system with carbs, you load it with sugar that immediately sends your body into hyperglycemia, that is, high levels of glucose in your blood.

This increase of blood glucose is normal, typically happening after a carb-heavy meal. As your body processes the glucose, sends it off to different tissues and organs, and stores the rest as fat, the concentration of sugar in your blood decreases.

After some time, the levels reach significantly low points, that put you in a state where your blood glucose levels are lower than normal.

What's the body's response? In an attempt to relieve the issue and to bring glucose back to normal levels, it activates cravings to make you hunger for carb-heavy food, knowing that that's what it takes to generate a quick spike in sugar once again.

That's why most people will crave for donuts, ice cream, and other sugary sweets, instead of things like vegetables and fruits, because the body knows where carbs come from.

On a carb-heavy diet, you'd be stuck in this endless cycle of hunger and cravings, because glucose isn't a stable macro that maintains relatively unchanged levels in your body. As it constantly dips and spikes, your body adjusts your response, to make sure you satisfy the needs that it detects.

This is all in pursuit of homeostasis - our body's tendency to work towards balance. With a fat-rich diet, the same doesn't apply.

The thing about stored fat is that it's highly available throughout the system, so there are lots of reserves to tap into. In the state of ketosis, your body won't need your deliberate action to supply macronutrients - it sources these itself by tapping into your stored fat.

So, there are no dips in energy availability, and thus no need to activate cravings. Other than that, fat itself can make people feel fuller and more satisfied for much longer after a meal.

Even during meal time, you might find yourself eating much less than you usually would on a carb-rich diet. This is another reason why counting calories might not be necessary on keto - because your body will send you the signals of satisfaction long before you even exceed your supposed calorie count.

Better Concentration

As one of the busiest organs in our system, brains consume over 50% of all carbohydrates consumed on a carb-rich diet. Unfortunately, long-term exposure to excess sugar can cause different types of neurological problems, including neurodegeneration.

What's more, gluten - a component typically found in carbohydrate-rich foods - may cause inflammation that impairs some neurological functions.

Before any of this happens though, you might find yourself experiencing fogginess of thought, memory, and cognition.

However, on a ketogenic diet, you're unlikely to experience any impairments to your concentration or attention span. This is because fat as an energy source can be much more efficient than glucose.

Each fat molecule provides more energy units per unit oxygen, so you get more fuel out of one fat molecule compared to one unit of glucose. On top of that, using fat as a main energy source for brain functions can increase the number of mitochondria in each brain cell.

These energy manufacturing centers on a cellular level are what fuel functioning on a microscopic level. In the brain, these power houses produce more cellular energy to fire up synapses and send neurological signals at a faster, more efficient rate.

All this considered, it's easy to see how you might experience better concentration, as your body enters a state of ketosis. Aside from being able to maintain your focus on a task much better, you might also notice overall improvement in other cognitive functions like memory, creativity, and analysis.

Weight Loss

As a mainstream diet, keto is peddled as one of the most effective weight loss strategies currently existing.

So many of those who attempt to observe it might be particularly interested in figuring out whether or not they've lost any weight after 3 weeks of dedicated effort.

The first thing you need to know however when measuring weight loss achieved through keto is that there is *no specific number* to expect. Everyone loses weight at different rates, so it really depends on how your body adapts to the change and how your body works in general.

Here are a few factors that could affect your weight loss:

Your Body Mass Index (BMI)

Your BMI is essentially a measurement of how much fat you have in relation to your height and weight.

For instance, take the case of two people who both weigh 160 lbs. Person A is just 5-feet tall, while person B nearly scrapes 6-feet.

Which person has more weight? Because height adds weight, the taller individual likely has much less fat than the shorter one.

There are categories of BMI, starting from underweight, to normal, to overweight, and obese.

Individuals who fall along the upper border of overweight, and within obese limits, typically have a harder time losing weight, and thus see less prominent results at the start.

Your Specific Fat Adaptation period

When you first begin your keto journey, you'll notice the opposite of all the supposed changes we've mentioned.

You might feel slow, sluggish, lacking in energy, and cloudy in thought. It's all a normal part of the process as your body learns to adjust and adapt to the new changes.

During the first few weeks of keto, your body will try to adapt to the sudden shift in energy supply. The prolonged state of ketosis will probably be new to your system, so it won't be quite as efficient when it comes to burning calories and fat stores.

If you're coming from a drastically different diet, such as a standard, carb-rich diet, you might find that it will take your body slightly longer to adapt to the change.

That said, you may not notice any weight differences as quickly as others on the same diet.

Your Level of Activity

As was mentioned a few chapters back, there are some things you can do to improve your metabolic rate and speed up the pace of weight loss during your diet.

However, since everyone adapts different exercise routines, it can be said that each person on the keto diet might experience varied rates of weight loss, depending on how active they are.

Put simply, the more you exercise, the faster you're likely to lose weight. The less you exercise, or the more sedentary your lifestyle is, the slower the weight loss.

Your Food Choices

Are you loading up on fatty junk food or making sure that you're choosing clean fat?

The quality of your food choices has a significant impact on your weight loss, because poor selections can slow down your metabolic rate.

Gobbling down junk food takes a toll on your body at the cellular level. These choices lack the micronutrients needed to fuel proper molecular functioning, thus causing minute processes to sputter and stall.

If you're unhealthy at the cellular level, you can expect that a number of your biological functions won't be at their best.

Your Health Status

How old are you? Do you have a history of disease or any pre-existing medical condition? Do you have vices like smoking?

Your overall health status will play a role in your weight loss. So trying to optimize it to accommodate better weight loss results, can produce more prominent changes sooner.

Some of the things you can change include cutting out vices, adopting a healthier sleeping schedule, and taking any medications and supplements, as recommended by your physician.

If you're suffering from any sort of condition that might have an effect on the rate of weight loss, be patient, observe treatment and management strategies, and ask your health care provider what you can do to achieve the best results with keto.

All of that said, there are some baseline weight loss numbers that you might be able to use to be able to set the proper expectations as you go along.

This can be broken down into weeks:

Week 1, Days 1-7

After the first week of observing the ketogenic diet, you can lose anywhere from 2 to 15 pounds, depending on the factors listed above.

This is probably the fastest drop you will achieve throughout the entire process, which can help improve your resolve to keep on going.

The reason for the sudden drop in weight isn't necessarily because of fat loss, but more likely because of water loss.

Each unit of glucose in your body is stored away with up to 3 units of water. These are tucked away in your muscles, ready to be used when the demand for energy is high. As you starve your body of carbs, it burns away excess glucose first, including those stored in the muscles.

As these units are used up, the water that bound them are now freed, and exit your system since there's no longer a need for them. This mass water loss can cause significant changes in your weight and might have you feeling less sluggish and bloated - both great to boost your dieting morale.

Of course, there might not be any apparent changes in terms of the way you look, but the takeaway when it comes to this specific change is that you have successfully started the journey to ketosis.

By encouraging your body to burn away the glucose stored in the muscles, you can assume that you have set ketosis in motion.

Over the next few weeks, you can expect to see even more changes in terms of your weight.

Week 2, Days 8-14

On the second week, you'll experience *fat adaptation*.

This basically pertains to your body's adjustment as it detects a change in your macronutrient consumption and alters its functionality to suit this new energy source.

So, while you might have felt sluggish, tired, slow, and cloudy at the start of your diet, during week 2, you'll notice all the positive changes starting to take form.

In terms of weight loss, any pounds you shed by this point will be a lot less drastic. So expect something more slow and steady.

By this time, you might be seeing a decrease of as little as 1lb to as much as 3.5lb, depending on your body's specific adaptation rate.

The better your body takes to the new diet, the faster your weight loss will be.

Week 3, Days 15-21

There might not be too much of a difference with the rate of weight loss between week 2 and 3, as long as you don't make any changes to your diet.

Loading up on quality food choices, adopting a healthy exercise routine, and trying out other tactics to boost your metabolism can have you losing between 1-3.5 lbs consistently.

Some studies have found that the rate of weight loss can remain unchanged for up to 3 months, after which it might start to slow down even further.

This is simply your body's natural tendency to maximize energy and make sure that it's not overspending fuel.

So, if all goes well and you're able to stick to the diet for 21 days, without making any mistakes in your method and while observing the right tactics towards boosting your metabolic rate, you might be able to achieve a total weight difference of up 17 to 22 lbs during the first 3 weeks.

Should you be aiming for weight loss that's much faster than that? According to experts - no.

Healthy weight loss shouldn't have you shedding pounds at lightning speed. Easing your body into the process and maintaining a slow, steady, consistent weight loss pace will help make the entire experience more rewarding and much safer for you.

It's important to keep in mind that weight loss results from the ketogenic diet are only possible when a specific circumstance is met - that is, ketosis.

Without ketosis, you wouldn't lose any weight. So, it's important to identify *if and when* your body enters the state of ketosis.

Here are a few tell-tale signs that signify that your ketogenic diet is bringing you to the right path:

Your breath stinks - well, it's not the most pleasant, but it does tell you you're doing things right. When you're deep into ketosis, your body releases different types of ketones. The specific one that affects your breath is called acetone, and it exits your body through your mouth and your urine.

While it might not be the most delightful issue to deal with, pear-drop smell or bad breath is a positive sign for your dietary efforts.

Just make sure if you're trying to keep that stinky stench at bay with mint candies and gum that you're not indulging in choices that incorporate too much sugar.

You're constipated or dehydrated - remember how during the first week, weight loss might be the result of a reduced water content in your system?

When this happens, it's not unlikely that you might feel dehydrated or constipated, due to a lack of fluid. So try to load up on more water by taking in a few extra glasses than you typically do.

For those who experience struggles with their bowel movements after the first week, a sugar-free electrolyte drink might be the best solution. Make sure to read labels first though, to make sure your chosen beverage isn't loading you up with unnecessary carbs.

You're having difficulty sleeping - insomnia is one of the earliest struggles you might face as you enter ketosis.

The sudden shift in energy source might make your brain sputter a little, interfering with some of the functions that it might have already mastered, before you made the change - like your sleep-wake pattern.

If you notice after you've started your ketogenic diet that you're having a little extra difficulty falling asleep at night, congratulations.

You've probably effectively started to burn away the last remaining glucose stores in your muscles, and your body is now searching for new resources to tap into.

You're having a bout of keto-flu - if you observed an excessively carb-heavy diet prior to making the change, you might experience what's called carb withdrawal.

LISA SCOTT

This is a period of adjustment that comes before fat adaptation, characterized by symptoms such as nausea, fatigue, headaches, and a dry mouth.

Collectively, these symptoms are called the 'keto-flu' and usually occur just a few days after you adapt to the diet.

Although they might not be the most pleasant effects to deal with, they do tell you that you've reached carbohydrate starvation. Any symptoms should subside over a few days and you should experience adaptation soon after.

If you notice that they persist, you might want to visit your physician for an expert opinion.

As with any other diet, try not to rush things and keep your efforts at a slow, steady, and safe pace. Any drastic changes that suddenly interrupt your body's normal functioning can be dangerous even over a short period of time.

So make sure to keep track of the signs and consult with your physician if you notice anything that might be a red flag.

5

COMMON KETO MISTAKES

We've all heard it before, *'I tried that fad keto diet before, it doesn't work'!*

Before you get discouraged by anecdotal sources telling you that the ketogenic diet won't work out for you, it's important to know that it's easier to make mistakes when observing the diet, than to follow through with keto guidelines.

Why? The answer is simple - lots of people don't read up, don't learn, and don't educate themselves on the proper execution of the keto diet. So, before you buy into those stories of failure, consider the fact that these people probably got it wrong, because they didn't do the research first.

Another way to keep yourself guarded from the pitfalls of keto, is to make sure you know all about them. Maintaining awareness. on the typical mistakes people make, can help you steer clear of them more efficiently as you maintain mindfulness on what you do and how you do it.

Failing to Achieve Ketosis

The very reason why the entire weight loss strategy is called the ketogenic diet is because it involves putting your body into a state of ketosis.

This metabolic stress urges your system to look for energy elsewhere as it senses depleted levels of carbohydrates and glucose, which is why it turns to tapping into fat storage that's accumulated in your muscles and tissues.

The goal of the game is to keep your body in a state of ketosis for as long as you're observing the diet. As long as ketosis continues, you will proceed to lose weight.

A few chapters back, it was discussed how you can detect whether you're in ketosis or not. If you've noticed though that you might not be *quite there* even days or weeks after you've began the change, then maybe you might want to consider these solutions.

Re-establish your Macros - the biggest reason why most people fail to maintain ketosis is because they eat *too many carbs.*

Even just stepping over the boundaries of your carb count by a few grams can provide your body enough glucose to run quite a few functions, kicking you out of the keto circle.

Try to take a step back and reassess your macro management methods. If you're taking in too many carbs, given the calories you consume, try to cut back even more. You might also want to consider the amount of protein you're eating. If you're chowing down on too much protein, relative to the amount of fat you're consuming, then you might struggle to shed the pounds.

Track Your Ketones - there are ways that you can track whether or not there's an excess of ketones in your system.

Local pharmacies usually sell tests that you can administer at home, using your breath, urine, or blood.

By measuring your ketones regularly, you can detect whether you're keeping your body in a state of ketosis, or whether you've stepped out.

In the case of the latter, you can re-establish your diet and calculate the amount of fat you're taking in, to re-enter ketosis.

Overlooking Hidden Carbs

In a perfect world, food packaging would give it to you straight. Unfortunately, it's not a perfect world.

Lots of food manufacturing and packaging companies keep a bunch of information off the labels or write their nutritional information in misleading ways.

The reason can be one or both of the following:

- Giving buyers a hard time understanding their labels can increase sales. That is, ignorance is bliss.

- Some products don't seem to need to provide nutritional information, so they're left out completely.

If you want to put your body in a state of ketosis, it's not enough to simply count the big carbs in your diet. Remember, *low carb might sometimes not be low enough* if you're aiming to achieve weight loss with the ketogenic diet.

Any excess can kick you out of ketosis and keep your system running on glucose for longer than you think. So, aside from keeping an eye out for carbs present in bread, pasta, rice, and other major meal components, consider how they might also be included in other ingredients, that you would have otherwise thought healthy.

For instance, *spices*. It's rare that you'll find any nutritional information of value on the packet of something like, garlic powder. But you'd be surprised to know that it can contain as much as 6 grams of carbs in every tablespoon. Add two tablespoons to your dish, and you've already got 12 grams in for your daily limit.

Spices, sauces, condiments, concentrates, extracts, and dressings - even some of those on the strictest ketogenic diets can overlook these products' labels because they seem too small and insignificant to count. But these things do add up, and they might just push you over your carb limit.

As a general rule, you should be more interested in whole foods, fresh vegetables and fruits, and foods that are as unprocessed as possible.

Even flavors and spices can be taken straight from the source, with a little research, so make sure you avoid buying into pre-packaged choices to steer clear of the excess carbs.

If you don't have any other choice, make sure you read up and plan ahead, to avoid adding too many carbs unknowingly.

The purpose of meal planning - aside from reducing the time you spend thinking about what to cook next - is to help you make informed choices, so that you don't end up consuming anything that doesn't fit your diet's parameters.

Taking in Too Many Calories

It's hard to go overboard when you're on a ketogenic diet, since fat tends to make you feel full sooner and longer.

So even if you previously had a voracious appetite before adapting the ketogenic diet, you might not be able to exceed your calorie limit in a day, if you're eating mostly fat.

Even then, there are some people who manage to eat more than they should while on keto. In any case, eating more than your body needs will lead to fat gain and storage, because it won't have anything else to do with the excess fat that you've consumed. If you're eating bad types of fat, your body can store it as plaque in your blood vessels or in your liver.

Aside from eating mostly fat, one of the main goals of keto weight loss is to eat just enough calories or less calories than what you need.

If you eat just enough, you achieve break-even and give your body some room to burn small amounts of fat storage at a time, since there isn't any excess left to store. If you eat less than you need, then you bump up fat burning, since your body needs to find fuel to fire up the different processes it performs.

Of course, there is a fine line between just the right deficit and too much deficit. Starving your body of both carbohydrates and calories can cause your metabolic rate to slow down completely and may be dangerous if observed for too long.

As a general rule, you should not aim for any more than a 500 calorie deficit, given your specific recommended caloric intake.

Most people think "1,200!" when they are confronted with the question of how many calories should I eat daily if I'm on a diet?

While that might sound right to most people, but in truth, there really is no magic number. Everyone is different, so deciding on the right caloric limit depends on your specific needs.

In one of the later chapters, we're going to be sharing everything you need to know about calculating your calories to meet your particular requirements, based on your weight, activity level, and also your fat percentage.

Eating Bad Fat

A few chapters back, we talked about the difference between good and bad fat.

On a keto diet, you will want to make sure you're still eating clean by indulging in more good fat, such as monounsaturated and polyunsaturated fats. These are fats that you can find in the food recommendations listed a ways back.

There are lots of different kinds of bad fat, like saturated fats, that you'll find in fast food, junk food, and basically poor food choices that don't really do well for long-term diets like keto.

The reason why they don't work is because they have no nutritional value to them. So loading up doesn't put your body in the best possible condition.

As with any other diet, you should be seeking to lose weight *and stay healthy* when you adopt a ketogenic diet. So fast food and junk food should still remain off of your menu if you want to get the best results out of your effort.

Remember, it's not enough to simply eat fat - you need to make sure that what you're eating is good quality fat that will help your body achieve optimal functioning, even at the cellular level.

Consuming Too Much Protein

One of the sneaky mistakes that people tend to commit on keto is eating too much protein.

On the surface, a person observing a keto diet might be more interested in cutting out carbs. This hyper vigilance and excessive awareness, directed towards carbohydrates, can make it easy to lose sight of proteins.

Remember, just like your carbs and fats, proteins are an energy source; they're macronutrients. So if you eat too much, you give your body yet another source of macros that it can use, aside from the fat you've already got stored.

Keep in mind that your body has a specific preference for fresh new macros that you consume and will choose to burn these before anything else because they're more readily available.

If you're eating too many proteins, relative to the amount of fats you're taking in, your body might choose to use up proteins first and keep the reserved fat in storage for later.

Mistaking Some Food as 'Keto'

No doubt, it's really not that easy to pinpoint *keto food* even if you read all the labels. After all, we can't all be expert nutritionists.

Unfortunately, dieters who have little to no experience when it comes to understanding the nutritional value and composition of food can make mistakes in the grocery store, thinking certain choices are keto, even if they're not.

Some of the most common mistakes people make involve vegetables, meats, and processed foods. For instance, many would think that 'meat is meat' and there really isn't anything else to consider when buying keto meat aside from its weight in grams. But a look into grass-fed and grain-fed specifics will tell you there's always more than meets the eye.

Grass-fed meat tends to be much richer in healthy fat and omega-3 and 6 fatty acids, making it a healthier, more appropriate choice for people on keto. Grain-fed meats on the other hand contain more calories. So 100 grams of grass-fed meat will give you more room in caloric intake compared to 100 grams of grain-fed meat.

Some vegetables have small amounts of carbohydrates that can add up easily. For instance, *onions* - a typical favorite flavor-adding ingredient - contains up to 6 grams of carbs for every 58 grams. If you add in even just half a cup into a salad or sautee, you end up with just around 24 carbs left before you hit your limit.

Make sure you do your research and maintain an awareness of how and where carbs can present themselves, so you don't end up stuffing your shopping cart with food choices that don't meet your keto needs.

Indulging Too Much in Snacks

The urge to snack might be significantly reduced when you assume a diet that's composed mostly of fat, since these macros tend to be more stable in your system, compared to glucose.

With reduced cravings and appetite, you might not find yourself fluttering in and out of the kitchen too often when it isn't meal time. Of course, it doesn't apply to *everyone*. There are some people who might still struggle with the urge to munch at odd hours.

Unfortunately during keto, watching your macros is an important part of achieving weight loss success. So you can't just grab a slice of cheese or a bunch of almonds and chew away to your heart's delight.

Unnecessary snacking can easily push you out of ketosis and put you over your caloric limit, so be careful.

If you've found that you still need to eat a few bites in between meals, consider planning your entire day's consumption before hand. This helps guide you towards making the right snack choices, and prevents eating any excess.

Keeping It Mental

There's nothing inherently wrong with keeping track of everything in your mind. But if you want to be accurate with all of your macros and other dietary practices, you might want to consider downloading a fitness app or investing some time into a fitness journal.

Keeping every last detail of your keto journey logged only in your head makes everything prone to error. Did you eat 300 grams or 450 grams? How many minutes did you actually work out? Are you really within your carb limit, or did you already exceed?

Of course, you can always answer these questions, based off of what you remember, but if you have a physical log, you can make much more precise corrections to your diet. The purpose of keeping information on your diet is to help you monitor your progress and make sure you're not doing anything that's counterproductive to your goals.

The "Tomorrow" Mentality

More often than not, you might find yourself falling off the wagon.

Maybe you ate too many carbs, maybe you didn't exercise today, maybe you chowed down on too many calories. Whatever the case, these minor slip-ups are a normal part of getting accustomed to a new diet, so there's no reason to beat yourself up over them.

They only become mistakes when you give up for the day and tell yourself you'll start again tomorrow.

This mentality often leads to a chain of new mistakes, causing you to binge, overindulge, and fall off the wagon even more.

Unfortunately, because of the delicate nature of ketosis, these seemingly harmless choices can make it difficult to get back on the horse.

If you slipped up, accept the error, dust off your shoulders, and get back on track. Correcting the mistake as soon as it's made minimizes its effects on your diet. However, choosing to go the other direction by saying you'll call the day a failure and just start again tomorrow, only brings you back to square one.

Guessing the Numbers

How many calories should you be aiming to consume in a day? What portion should be dedicated to carbohydrates, to proteins, and to fats?

Lots of people feel that they can guess the numbers and still get the same results. After all, if it's mostly fat, it's gotta be keto, right?

While that might seem like sound reasoning, it's important to remember that your body runs on specific macronutrients and it's very possible to feed it all the wrong stuff, if you're not completely aware of what it needs.

There are lots of anecdotal sources that spread information about failed keto attempts, saying the diet is nothing more than a fad. But more often than not, these individuals didn't really crunch the numbers before starting, so ketosis was never achieved.

- Weigh yourself

- count your calories, and

- figure out your base metabolic rate

These are all essential numbers that should help you figure out the proper macronutrient portions when you start cooking up those keto meals.

Of equal importance, you should try to familiarize yourself with the specific macronutrient profiles for the food you buy. Knowing this information will help you understand whether the food you've chosen really is keto or just seems like it.

Staying on Keto for Too Long

If you thought you could observe the keto diet as a lifelong dietary plan to reduce fat and maintain your new figure, it's important to note that the ketogenic diet wasn't designed for long-term observance.

If anything, keto makes a great solution if you're looking for a weight loss method that provides fast results over a short period of time. After a few weeks on keto, it's important that you seek out a more sustainable diet that suits your nutritional needs and helps maintain the weight loss you've achieved.

That's why you'll find a chapter on intermittent fasting later in this book, it's the perfect accompaniment to the keto diet, for maintaining the weight you've just lost.

Why shouldn't keto be used as a long-term diet plan? It's simple - ketosis isn't a state that your body should be in for too long.

Remember, the state of ketosis is your body's response to metabolic stress. There isn't enough glucose in your system, so it looks for other sources it can use to fuel your different functions.

In layman's terms, ketosis is starvation. So, despite eating a full load of calories every day, your body interprets that your current dietary situation is the result of you starving.

In the long run, you might start to feel too much fatigue, you may experience muscle loss, and perhaps even develop a dangerous condition called ketoacidosis. When there's a proliferation of ketones in your body over a long period of time, your internal environment becomes acidic.

This change in your pH balance - if sustained over a prolonged period - can be dangerous to liver, kidney, and brain. In some cases, ketoacidosis has been found to cause irreversible organ damage and even death.

Another thing you might want to consider, is the fact that the keto diet isn't necessarily a well-balanced diet.

Of course, those carbs can be nasty for your weight. If you consider all the angles, it's easy to see that these macronutrients, as well as a number of micronutrients, that you can only consume through certain restricted food choices, are an important facet of a healthy diet.

By cutting out food groups entirely and limiting your choices to just fatty foods, you pave the way for nutritional deficiencies.

Unfortunately, there is no way to completely discount the value and importance of glucose in our system. That's why many of the staple foods around the world mainly use glucose - because it's the ideal energy source to fuel our different biological functions.

Without glucose, everything will reach an all-time low - from your weight, to your muscle mass, your electrolytes, and yes, even your blood pressure and blood glucose.

Sure, low levels of blood glucose might be ideal if you're predisposed to diabetes or if you already have it, but for healthy, disease-free individuals, hypoglycemia can cause a host of problem in the long run, including seizures, problems in consciousness, and visual disturbances. Chronic hypotension on the other hand, can be equally dangerous, putting individuals at risk of fainting spells.

Finally, it's also worth mentioning that fat can become plaque in the blood vessels. If you have a family history of heart disease, a build up of atherosclerotic plaque can lead to a variety of cardiovascular conditions that might plague you for the rest of your life.

This is particularly possible for those who indulge too much in poor food choices, that incorporate the wrong types of fat as well as low-density lipoproteins.

Experts recommend that individuals observe the keto diet for no more than 3 to 4 months. Extending beyond that could give rise to poor weight loss outcomes and may be more dangerous to your health, than beneficial.

6

MAKING THE MOST OF THE KETO DIET

The ketogenic diet was first created and tested by Dr. Gianfranco Cappello, an associate doctor of surgery at the Sapienza University.

During the initial trial of his research, he claimed that the keto diet was able to show successful results for an astonishing 19,000 participants.

The dieters participating in the study experienced significant, rapid weight loss, and were able to maintain their new figure, even after one year had passed.

Whilst the overall method used during his research varies greatly from the way the keto diet is used in the mainstream setting today, the principles remain pretty much the same, and dieters can expect similar outcomes.

If there's one thing worth mentioning though, it's that Cappello did emphasize that the keto diet was best for quick bursts of weight loss over a short period of time.

He developed the diet to be used for aggressive fat reduction achieved within a short time frame, so the keto diet really isn't ideal as a permanent dietary plan.

The reason why many people try to sustain keto as a prolonged method of weight loss, is because of the fear of weight gain. Of course, your body will become fat adapted, so introducing glucose once again at the end of a ketogenic diet cycle, might result in weight gain.

Fortunately however, Cappello was able to prove that weight loss can be kept off, as a majority of his participants demonstrated.

During the 1 year post-diet check-up, it was found that patients had a mean weight gain of 15.4% - a very modest number considering the fact that the keto diet was completely ceased and most of the patients didn't employ any weight loss or maintenance tactics, after ending the study.

While that might seem promising, there are a few things you can do to help maintain your weight loss. These strategies should help you keep the weight off, and maintain your healthy, new physique, even after the keto journey has ended.

For one solution to maintaining weight loss, check out chapter 8. We'll look at the different types of intermittent fasting, which can really help you to keep off the weight that you've lost on the keto diet.

Maintain a Healthy Lifestyle

A sedentary lifestyle that doesn't involve a lot of exercise or physical activity is one of the cornerstones of weight gain.

If you're hoping to keep the weight off after you've stopped observing keto, you might want to consider adapting a healthier lifestyle, to keep your metabolism fired up.

Daily routines, that account for no more than 30 minutes of your time, can be more than enough to keep that extra weight from creeping back onto your body.

Cardio exercises can be easy and practical for maintenance, but since you're probably consuming more carbs and proteins after keto, you might also want to incorporate some weight lifting into your repertoire.

Heavy lifting and high intensity workouts, that are demanding on your body, will burn more calories not only immediately after the workout, but also as you go throughout your day.

So, if you'd still be burning calories up to 8 hours after a jog, you could burn calories for as much as 24 hours after heavy weight lifting.

Keep Calories in Check

If you eat more calories than you burn, you will gain weight. That's just one of the basics.

So, if you want to make sure that you're keeping the weight off, you should be careful not to eat more calories than your body needs in a day.

Do you need to create a major deficit to achieve weight maintenance? Not exactly. Staying within the ideal limit can be good enough.

So, if your calculations tell you that you should consume a total of 1800 calories a day to meet your caloric needs, you can stick to that. You can create a minor deficit with your exercise or by taking out a small number, if you really want to be on the safe side.

Eat Clean

Just as you're encouraged to indulge in healthy keto food, you should also make it a point to observe a clean diet once you're off of ketosis.

Healthy, whole foods that come as close to the source as possible are always the best. So try to avoid anything packaged, canned, or processed. Healthy food choices help improve your overall wellness and keep your body working in tip top shape.

As a general rule, you should still aim to steer clear of junk food, sugary sweets and treats, and fast food since they never really provide any nutritional value whatever diet you might be on.

On top of that, you might also want to consider the way you prep your meals. Choosing healthy recipes that incorporate all the different essential food groups can give you balanced nutrition. Include vegetables and fruits into your diet, and make sure to eat just enough meat, along with your daily intake of carbs.

You might also want to opt for cooking methods that use less oil, such as roasting or boiling ,to get the highest nutritional value from your chosen foods.

To make sure you're really investing in your health, it's also ideal that you consider taking in multivitamins or supplements, that can help fill in the gaps that might be present in your diet.

Even individuals who are particularly mindful of eating only healthy, whole foods are likely to miss out on a few micronutrients, so try to find the gap and fill it in with a trusted supplement.

Rotate Your Diets

One strategy that many keto dieters apply to help keep their weight off is diet rotation.

That is, after completing one cycle of keto for a few months, they shift to a standard diet. After sticking to that for a while, they shift back to keto, just to shed off any extra pounds they might have gained on their standard diet.

Cyclical dieting is great, because it allows your body to revert back to non-starvation status, without losing the inherent benefits of low blood glucose and HDLs. So consider switching your diet back and forth over a given period of time. For instance, some keto dieters shift diets 4 times a year, rotating between keto and their standard diet every 3 months.

There are also other versions of keto that are worth taking a look into. Cycle keto entails going onto keto for 6 days a week, and then reserving 1 day as your cheat day when you either eat a standard diet, or slightly more carbs than you typically would.

This helps refresh your system and makes sure that you're getting just enough of all the macros and micros you need in a week. The issue of course is that that single cheat day can kick you out of ketosis and cause you to even store glucose if you dedicate yourself to eating too much of it over the 24 hour period.

The problem, of course, is that once you do indulge in even just slightly more carbohydrates, you end up having to deal with hunger pangs and cravings all over again.

So, the start of every new week as you restart your keto diet, after the cheat day can be exceptionally difficult, because you disrupt your body as it closes in on fat-adaptation.

Of course, there are some who question its efficacy. And somehow, the fact that it doesn't really have that much scientific research to back it up can make it slightly less reliable. Even so, it might be worth a shot.

Small Frequent Meals

Once you start to balance out your macros again, you might start to feel hunger pangs and cravings more frequently once more.

This is your body's natural response to the influx of glucose which you might not be able to avoid on a standard diet. Of course, it's okay to give in every now and then. But it's also easy to fly off the handle and eat way more than you're supposed to.

To help keep your cravings and your hunger at bay, consider dividing your meals into 5 smaller portions that are regularly scheduled during your waking hours - one for breakfast, one for lunch, one in the late afternoon, one for dinner, and one after dinner.

The purpose of small frequent meals is to help you manage your calories, so that you get the same amount of food at different points throughout the day. The schedule keeps you from feeling hungry and reaching into your fridge for snacks that fall outside of your supposed caloric intake.

Divide the number of calories you eat by 5. That should give you a solid figure to work off of, so you can structure your meals to fall within the proper caloric limits. So if you eat 1800 calories in a day, each meal should be a maximum of 360 calories.

Stay On Top

While there are a large number of keto dieters that are afraid of losing their results after reverting back to their standard diet, there are those who feel too confident with their outcomes.

That is, they feel like the weight loss will definitely stay off, so there's no need to keep an eye on their progress, after their keto journey has ended.

Unfortunately, failing to stay on top of changes is the primary reason for weight gain. When it comes to weight management, it's always easier to gain than lose fat, so even the slightest mistakes after keto can make a big difference on your loss and bring you right back to square one.

To avoid this, you should make it a point to stay on top of your progress. Monitor your weight, keep a journal, and schedule regular exercise routines to stay on track.

You'll find that it's easier and better if you plan your meals ahead and pattern your grocery store choices after the meal plans you've created. This prevents you from stocking up on food that might end up as excess or go to waste, and helps guarantee that what you eat in a day is exactly what you need - no more, no less.

Forget Cheat Day

Consider this - you've successfully completed 3 months of keto and lost 22 pounds during the process.

You've now adapted a new standard diet that puts you at your 1700 caloric limit in a day. You don't eat in excess of what you need and stay dedicated to your boundaries to prevent weight gain.

At the end of every week however, you indulge in one cheat day during which you eat an average of 600 calories more than you actually need.

Will you gain weight? The short answer is yes - you most certainly will.

When you eat just enough calories to meet your needs, you reach breakeven. This simply means that there isn't a deficit between the calories you eat and the calories you burn, and there isn't an excess either. This is great for weight maintenance, because it doesn't call for storage and doesn't burn anything other than your intake.

On that single cheat day, when you allow yourself to eat 600 calories, you end up consuming 600 more than your daily limit.

If you're not doing anything to offset this - such as exercise - the extra intake will be stored as fat. And since you're only aiming for breakeven for the rest of the week, you're unlikely to burn the extra 600 calories any other day.

Cheat day is a major pitfall for most people, thinking it's something that anyone and everyone can indulge in, without incurring any damage to their weight loss.

The fact remains however that the concept of cheat day really only applies to individuals that have successfully established an aggressive exercise routine.

Heavy weight lifters, gym buffs, and athletes can comfortably indulge in extra calories any day of the week because their bodies are well-adjusted, burning calories more rapidly than most standard dieters.

Sleep More and Stress Less

Studies have found a link between poor sleeping habits and weight gain, and even tag it as one of the major contributors to obesity.

Getting a full 8 hours of uninterrupted, quality sleep at night can significantly boost metabolism and promote healthier habits during your waking hours.

Individuals who observe proper sleeping routines have been found to eat less, move more, and make better dietary choices throughout the day. So they're far less prone to gaining weight compared to those with impaired sleeping practices.

Another thing you might want to consider is how you manage your stress. According to studies, stress has been found to be a major reason for overeating, since most people seem to draw comfort and relief from consuming sugary sweets and carb-loaded treats.

Practicing the proper stress management techniques can help reduce the number of calories you consume in a day.

Calming strategies, meditation, and deep breathing are just some of the alternatives you can take in place of gobbling down a tub of ice cream when you start to feel the heat.

Get Support

Weight loss and weight management are two tasks that are made easier with the help of friends - so make sure you get some well-deserved support.

Having someone with you who's out to achieve the same goals can make it much more difficult to fall off the wagon, since you've got a little extra motivation.

What's more, working with a friend to achieve weight management makes it easier to get back on track, if you find yourself straying away from your proper path.

Work out together, plan meals together, and keep each other updated on your success and even your failures. Don't be afraid to be honest with one another - failure to meet some of the parameters of your new diet shouldn't be shameful.

Aim to comfort each other during times of failure and uplift one another to get back on the wagon after a bad day. Being accountable to someone else is a really great way to help you stay on track.

Another way you might want to get support is by finding online groups and forums, where dieters discuss their progress. Social media platforms are an excellent example of places where you can find like-minded individuals on the same journey.

Applications for tracking your progress, your meals, and your exercise also have like-minded communities where you can share information on how your diet is getting along.

Maintaining a presence on these types of platforms makes it much easier to commit to your new diet. Herd mentality improves a person's resolve to stay on track, especially because there are many others who can inspire you with their progress and personal experiences.

The ability to share information on your own journey can also amp up your desire to keep going, so try to find people or communities that allow you to talk about how far you've come.

Try Intermittent Fasting

Intermittent fasting is another dietary technique that's becoming more and more popular throughout the world.

The basic principle behind it is that it helps individuals lose weight by tossing the body into a state of starvation at certain points throughout the day. So unlike the ketogenic diet which calls for a continuous state of ketosis, intermittent fasting breaks it up into phases. One phase of the day is for eating, and the other is for fasting.

Lots of keto dieters have adopted the intermittent fasting schedule into their standard diet, because it helps maintain a pseudo-starvation state for a short period of time.

In the long run, intermittent fasting can be much less dangerous, since it does allow the consumption of other macronutrients.

The challenge lies in the willpower needed to see through the fasting hours. Unlike keto, intermittent fasting calls for a long period of time during which an individual shouldn't eat anything.

This period of fasting is what bumps up the metabolic processes that fuel the burning of calories. Sure, it's really not that easy to maintain yourself without food for a long period of time, especially if you're experiencing hunger pangs and cravings. But with a little practice and discipline, it is possible to get done.

Just like any diet however, the intermittent fasting technique comes with its own fair share of downsides. For instance, because everyone burns calories at a different pace, the fasting window might not be long enough for some individuals, calling for the need to extend the phase without food, to make sure that any excess would be burnt, before the intake of any new macronutrients.

Another cause for concern is the fact that it allows the intake of carbs, which simply means that hunger pangs and cravings may be significantly pronounced during the fasting hours.

This makes it more difficult to avoid sneaking into the kitchen to break the fast before time is up. Nonetheless, it is possible to adapt to the intermittent fasting schedule with ease.

Taking it slowly and trying to ease yourself into the process, instead of jumping in head first, should make the transition far less taxing on your body.

It's also recommended that you curtail your intake of carbs. While you can eat more carbs than you would on keto, eating slightly less carbohydrates than the standard diet entails, will help keep cravings at bay during intermittent fasting.

LISA SCOTT

7

21-DAY DIET PLAN

Twenty-one days.   That's all you really need to get the most out of your ketogenic diet journey.

The strategy was developed for aggressive weight loss, so dieters don't really need to go overboard by observing its parameters all year round.

The beauty of the ketogenic diet is that it provides quick results for fast gratification, making it easier to stay on track for the three weeks required to win your body back. The question now is - how exactly can you apply it to your life to get the results you want?

Throughout this guide, it was mentioned time and time again that everyone is different. So although the ketogenic diet works for most, if not all, of those who try it out, minute tweaks to the general concept can help make it even more effective for your specific needs.

To help you answer that question, we've put together this ultimate guide on how you can adjust and adapt the ketogenic diet, to create your very own 21-day plan to suit your particular lifestyle and preferences.

Step 1 - Understanding Your Body

The first thing you need to do in order to plan your very own ketogenic journey would be to determine your body's unique specifications.

By figuring out the details of your system, you can get calculate more accurate numbers when planning your macros, your exercise routine, and the portions of your meals.

As with any diet, the very first thing you need to do before you begin keto is to weigh yourself. This number will set the stage for all of your other efforts and give you a solid understanding of where you currently stand, so you can manage your expectations for the rest of the diet.

Here are a few tips to getting an accurate measurement of your weight:

- Make sure your weighing scale is properly calibrated and placed on a level surface

- Weigh yourself every day for a week before you begin your diet

- Wear as little clothing as possible

- Step on the scale in the morning after you've gone to the bathroom

- Stand still and try to make sure that your weight is distributed evenly across the surface of the scale

Take your weight, once a day, every morning for a week, before you begin your diet. Once you've got a week's worth of data, compute the average. This should be your working weight measurement. All other computations should use this number as your weight.

Make sure you've got your weight measured in kilograms. If it's in pounds, just divide it by 2.2.

Now that you have an accurate weight measurement, it's time to compute your body fat percentage. This is an essential variable in determining how many calories you should be consuming in a day.

While tests that use measuring tape might be easier and faster, those that use body fat calipers are far more accurate. With an accuracy rating of +/- 3 percent error rate, this is the most reliable home test you can perform to get a good idea of your body fat percentage.

Here are some of the things you'll need to properly accomplish the Jackson and Pollock three-site formula for measuring body fat with calipers:

- Calipers

- An assist

- Measuring tape

- Marker

- Pen and paper

The calipers you purchased should have usage instructions included in the package. Make sure to read the directions, to guarantee proper and accurate usage and results.

If they didn't, here are a few tips on how to properly use them.

- Calipers are most accurate when used at eye level, so to make sure you've got the right measurements, enlist the help of an assistant.

- Test the pinch, by pinching the excess skin over the testing site with your index finger and thumb. Make sure you've got as much flesh between your fingers as possible, to get the appropriate reading. Pinching less fat or skin than what is available will cause inaccurate readings.

- Place the calipers' pinchers just a centimeter above your fingers, pinching your skin. Make sure to clamp as much of the excess skin's density with your calipers.

- Take the reading twice or thrice if you want to be sure of the measurements you've collected.

- Have a paper and pen at the ready, to record your readings.

For men, the three site method collects data from these locations:

- Chest

- Abdomen

- Thigh

For women, these are the testing sites:

- Triceps

- Suprailiac (that's just above the hip)

- Thigh

Once you have the measurements, you have the option to punch the numbers into an online calculator for Jackson and Pollock body fat percentage computations, or you can crunch the numbers yourself.

It's recommended that you find a reliable online calculator,   since the computation itself is prone to errors, if you're not as experienced with the process. With this number, you can now find out your 'lean factor multiplier'.

This number is what experts use to get an accurate numerical representation of your basal metabolic rate.

MALE		FEMALE	
Body fat percentage	Lean factor multiplier	Body fat percentage	Lean factor multiplier
10-14	1.0	14-18	1.0
15-20	0.95	19-28	0.95
21-28	0.9	29-38	0.9
Over 28	0.85	Over 38	0.85

Now, by this point, you should have both your weight in kilograms and your lean factor multiplier (LFM). You now have two of three variables needed to compute your basal metabolic rate. The third and last variable is simply your gender - which is 1.0 for males and 0.9 for females.

To compute your basal metabolic rate (BMR), follow this formula:

BMR = weight x gender x 24 x LFM

Applied, the numbers would look something like this:

BMR = 64 kgs x 0.9 x 24 x 0.9

BMR = 1,244.16

Now, after all that, you might be wondering - what was the point of all that math? The answer is simple - your basal metabolic rate represents the amount of calories you would burn if you were to lie down at home, doing nothing all day long.

This is what your body will naturally, effortlessly burn, day in and day out, to make sure all of the different functions of your body are adequately and properly performed.

While all of those numbers might seem like a mouthful already, it's important that you factor in your level of activity to figure out just how much you really need to get you through the day.

Remember, your BMR represents calories used for zero physical exertion, which is unrealistic even if you work a sedentary desk job.

Consider these Activity Level Multipliers:

Numerical Value	Description
1.3 (Very light)	Traditional office work or student lifestyle (sitting at a desk, minimal physical exertion, a few minutes of walking every day, mostly during the commute)
1.55 (Light)	Workers that walk around during work hours, such as teachers, store managers, and waiters)
1.65 (Moderate)	Employment or household work that calls for significant physical activity such as cleaning, landscaping, and home improvement. Individuals who jog or walk 15-30 minutes 3 days a week are included.
1.8 (Heavy)	Heavy manual labor including those working in construction, or athletes. Individuals who work out in the gym 3 or more days a week are included.
2.0 (Very heavy)	Minimum 8 hours of daily heavy manual labor. Individuals who work out 5 days or more and dedicate most of their time to fitness are included.

Take your BMR and multiply it to your activity level multiplier.

Based on the example provided above, we can come up with this example, for a moderately active person:

Daily Caloric Need = 1,244.16 x 1.65 = 2,052.86

To help you bump up your weight loss, you can subtract between 300 - 400 calories, to create a deficit in your daily intake. So instead of 2,052.86 calories, you might consume just 1753.86. This is still a reasonable amount, albeit less than your daily needs.

Do you need to incorporate a deficit? Not in all cases. Remember that everyone is different, so while some people might benefit from a caloric deficit, others might not.

Those who adapt healthy lifestyles, who exercise regularly, who have jobs that require quite a lot of physical exertion might not need the deficit since they're more likely to burn through what they eat.

Those who have a sedentary lifestyle, who don't necessarily workout regularly, and who have jobs that call for very little physical activity would benefit more from the deficit given that they might not be doing a lot to burn what they consume.

From here, we move on to step 2.

Step 2 - Managing Your Macros

Now that you know exactly how many calories you need in a day, you can start to create a pattern for your future portions, so you can make the right choices when planning out your meals. This is called managing your macros.

Macros are divided into three main categories - fats, carbs and proteins. Making sure that you're eating just enough of each is one of the cornerstones of the ketogenic diet, so it's important to get the numbers right.

According to experts, your keto diet should be made up of - up to 80% fat, 15% protein, and 5% carbohydrates.

The grams per macro changes depending on the number of calories you should consume in a day, which is why it's important to make sure you've got the right calorie computation.

For instance, a person who's supposed to consume around 1,450 calories a day, should have the following macro break down:

- 30 grams net carbs (after fiber is subtracted)

- 53 grams of protein

- 125 grams of fat

How were these numbers reached?

For protein, it's pretty simple - just 1 gram per every kilo of body weight. If you weigh 60 kilos, you need a maximum of 60 grams of protein.

For carbs, experts recommend bare minimum, at just 5-10% of your daily caloric intake. So in most cases, the carbs you consume will come from added ingredients like spices, seasonings, and some vegetables.

Fat on the other hand, should be the main component of your macro intake, at around 80% of your daily caloric limit.

Because it can be tough to manually compute these numbers, it's recommended that you download a reliable application or seek out an online macro calculator, to help you get the most precise numbers possible.

As a general rule, you should be eating below 50 grams of carbohydrates in a day, with your protein at par with your weight in kilos. All that's left should be composed of nothing other than fat.

Use these central principles when cooking up your meal plans, and you'd likely achieve ketosis after a day or two.

Step 3 - Meal Prep

The most fun you'll have with the ketogenic diet is probably in the kitchen.

Choosing ingredients and cooking meals can make it exceptionally exciting. But because not everyone can be a kitchen whiz, it's easy to feel confused and clumsy during those first few steps into keto-hood.

So you might be wondering - what makes a suitable keto meal?

Here's a sample 21-day meal guide to give you a better idea of what you can cook up:

Day 1
Breakfast - Bacon and eggs
Lunch - Pork sausage with avocado buns
Dinner - Eggs and vegetables stir-fry

Day 2
Breakfast - Baked eggs with vegetables and yogurt
Lunch - Shrimp cauliflower rice
Dinner - Chicken liver steak

Day 3

Breakfast - Smoked salmon and egg-stuffed avocado

Lunch - Creamy mashed cauliflower with keto gravy

Dinner - Cheesy beef patties

Day 4

Breakfast - Cauliflower and vegetable fritters

Lunch - Beef, eggs, and avocado salad

Dinner - Crabmeat-stuffed mushrooms with cream cheese filling

Day 5

Breakfast - Bacon, egg, and spinach flourless breakfast muffins

Lunch - Spicy shrimp and spinach omelette

Dinner - Ground beef tacos with cream cheese and crispy cheese shells

Day 6

Breakfast - Keto pancakes, made with almond flour

Lunch - Cheesy zucchini with bacon and eggs

Dinner - Beef and broccoli stir fry

Day 7

Breakfast - Mozzarella, turkey sausage, and bell pepper breakfast bake

Lunch - Creamy shrimp and salmon skillet

Dinner - Cauliflower and bacon mashed hash

Day 8

Breakfast - Bacon-wrapped avocado fries

Lunch - Zucchini grilled cheese sandwiches

Dinner - Tossed vegetables with cheese and olive oil

Day 9

Breakfast - Bacon, blue cheese, and chives devilled eggs

Lunch - Pan seared salmon with lemon and cream cheese

Dinner - Creamy chicken breast with bacon strips and cheese

Day 10

Breakfast - Keto cauliflower crust breakfast pizza

Lunch - Spinach, chorizo, and goat cheese omelette

Dinner - Tomato and feta cheese soup

Day 11

Breakfast - Kale and mushroom pork patties

Lunch - Hard-boiled egg-stuffed ground beef balls

Dinner - Mashed cauliflower with grilled shrimp

Day 12

Breakfast - Cauliflower and bacon stir fry

Lunch - Avocado and sausage egg casserole

Dinner - Smoked salmon and cream cheese on crunchy zucchini crusts

Day 13

Breakfast - Prosciutto wrapped asparagus with soft boiled eggs

Lunch - Kale, bacon, and mushroom egg wraps

Dinner - Sardine, artichoke, and egg pot pies

Day 14

Breakfast - Chicken, bacon, and zucchini stuffed avocado boats

Lunch - Pork belly and kimchi stir fry

Dinner - Spinach and cream cheese stuffed chicken breasts

Day 15

Breakfast - Crunchy cauliflower breadsticks

Lunch - Chicken satay with peanut sauce

Dinner - Lemon butter baked salmon

Day 16

Breakfast - Denver omelette salad

Lunch - Deconstructed fish tacos

Dinner - Sauteed cucumber thins with cheese

Day 17

Breakfast - Coconut flour breakfast crepes

Lunch - Tossed shrimp and avocado chunks in olive oil

Dinner - Blue cheese pork medallions

Day 18

Breakfast - Cream cheese cinnamon pancakes

Lunch - Spiced beef burgers with buttered vegetables

Dinner - Sage-rubbed baked salmon

Day 19

Breakfast - Spicy tuna and egg omelette

Lunch - Roasted cauliflowers with lemon butter sauce

Dinner - Bacon-wrapped beef and cheese patties

Day 20

Breakfast - Sausage breakfast burger with scrambled eggs and avocado

Lunch - Chicken and broccoli in dill sauce

Dinner - Spicy stir fried pork with cauliflower rice

Day 21

Breakfast - Bacon, egg, and spinach-stuffed bell peppers

Lunch - Salmon and avocado nori roll ups

Dinner - Sauteed salmon, mushrooms, and goat cheese

And there you have it!

Upon completing this easy meal prep guide, you would have successfully completed the 21-day keto diet and lost those extra pounds that have been pestering you.

Of course, portion size matters, and it's recommended that you take your caloric requirements into account when deciding how much of each meal you should eat.

One of the things you'll notice about this meal plan is that it doesn't complicate things, especially right off the bat.

Your first breakfast is really just your run-of-the-mill bacon and eggs - no elaborate preparation, no fancy bells and whistles.

If you're planning to develop your own meal plan, consider adapting to this principle - keep it simple.

A major deal-breaker for dieters especially as the initial excitement of adopting a new diet takes the back seat, is the effort and time it takes to prepare food. A high maintenance diet is unlikely to stick around, even if it's only intended to last 21 days.

Unless you're fully invested in spending your time in the kitchen and coming up with new recipes, consider planning simpler meals. This should help make it easier to stay dedicated to your diet, and prevent you from tapping out when you feel like there's just too much effort involved.

If you're wondering what you can have for snacks, consider these suggestions.

- Guacamole and zucchini sticks

- Pork rinds

- Baked flourless breadless keto onion rings

- Peanut butter and celery sticks

- Peanut butter and pecan candy bark

- Fudgy carb-free fat bombs

- Hard-boiled eggs

- Seaweed

- Deli meat and cheese roll ups

- Mixed nuts

- Beef jerky

- Crunchy sea salt kale chips

- Caprese salad

Step 4 - Lifestyle Check

The way to make sure your keto efforts are taking you where you want to go is to check the rest of your lifestyle.

There's more to weight loss than just eating specific kinds of food. Optimizing sleep, micronutrient intake, water consumption, and stress levels are just some of the other important facets of effective fat loss.

Water Intake

Remember that during the first week, a lot of the weight you'll lose will be due to water loss.

Glucose binds to water molecules when stored in the muscles, so when they're burnt away as you enter ketosis, you end up with less water in your system.

This can lead to dehydration and constipation. During the first 7 days of your keto journey, you need to make sure that you drink at least 2 liters of water a day. Some experts even suggest drinking more than that, gulping down a glass of water, even when you're not thirsty.

After the first week, drinking 2 or more liters of water is still recommended. This helps curb constipation, hunger and dehydration, as your body adapts to the drastic dietary change.

Micronutrients

In the long run, the ketogenic diet can become the cause of micronutrient deficiencies and malnutrition.

Over the short term though, early signs of gaps in your micronutrient profile can cause disturbances in the way you feel. Closing these gaps with multivitamins and supplements can help ease the side-effects of change and keep you on track to the end of your 21-day journey.

Aside from eating whole foods like vegetables, fruits, and fresh meats, consider taking a multivitamin or a supplement, to help make sure you're really meeting your body's needs for vitamins and minerals.

According to experts, some of the most affected micronutrients on the keto diet include sodium, potassium, B vitamins, calcium, iron, phosphorus, vitamins A and C, and zinc. Seeking out vitamins and supplements that offer these micronutrients can help make it possible for you to achieve optimal health even in ketosis.

Sleep

A lack of sleep has been closely linked with weight gain and obesity. Sleeping routinely on a predictable schedule and getting enough nighttime sleep every night can help boost your metabolism and increase the rate of your weight loss.

Before your body becomes fat-adapted, you will notice some problems with sleep. Insomnia is one of the more frustrating side effects of the ketogenic diet, this is usually due to a sign of magnesium deficiency, especially because during those first few days, you might feel more hunger and cravings. This, combined with sleeplessness, makes for a formidable opponent against your willpower to fight the urge to snack in the early hours.

Some experts suggest taking supplements that help ease insomnia. Be careful though - some formulations tend to sneak in a few carbs and sugars that make them non-keto friendly. That said, you might want to consider loading up on dinner just a few hours before you hit the hay, if you're not keen on taking supplements. This should help induce drowsiness, so you feel sleepier when night time hits.

Stress

When people are stressed, they tend to eat more. Even if you're on keto, eating in excess of your caloric needs can cause weight gain, especially if you go overboard drastically too often.

Managing your stress to improve your eating habits can make it easier to stick to your meal plans and avoid eating off schedule.

Practicing mindfulness, deep breathing, and heading out for a well-deserved spa treatment at the end of every week can help reduce stress and boost your metabolism. This also decreases the chances of getting grabby in the kitchen, when you've already reached your maximum caloric limit for the day.

Exercise

How much exercise is enough exercise? How do you know if you're doing enough to boost your metabolism and thus your fat loss? Are you doing the right kind of exercises, given the fat-intensive diet you're on?

As a general rule, any physical activity is better than no activity.

People tend to think that there are specifics they need to observe if they want to properly exercise while on keto. And while it is true that there might be some guidelines, the specifics aren't set in stone.

Performing a few minutes of cardio a day can be substantial enough to improve the results you get out of your ketogenic diet. Then again, opting to walk to your office, instead of taking your car, can also be a suitable adjustment to help you burn off the extra pounds.

Just keep in mind though that, since fat isn't that easily accessible to our system as a macronutrient, it takes quite a bit of time before we can tap into it for intense workouts. So heavy lifting, working with gym equipment, and hard physical exercise like mountain climbing can be more dangerous than beneficial.

Choose to stick to light intensity, low impact cardio workouts such as jogging, biking, and swimming. You might also want to consider longer distances instead of faster paces since your body will only tap into fat reserves after around 2 minutes of continuous physical exertion.

8

KEEPING OFF THE WEIGHT WITH INTERMITTENT FASTING

So, you've successfully managed to achieve your target weight with your ketogenic diet journey.

Now it's time to adapt to a new diet, to help your body adjust from ketosis back to a healthier long-term weight management strategy.

Sure, there are a lot of available options out there. But many of those who have gone through keto claim that intermittent fasting is the ideal weight management solution, for those who really want to keep the pounds off.

As the name suggests, intermittent fasting involves restricting your meals to a specific time frame, and then fasting for the rest of the day.

Unlike most other diets, intermittent fasting doesn't put a lot of weight on your dietary choices. Instead, it emphasizes the importance of your diet schedule.

If you come to think of it, you might already be observing fasting with your usual diet. Sleeping is a period of time during which you don't take in any calories and can be considered a fasting phase.

With intermittent fasting, you simply extend that period to cover a longer span of time. At the start, it might feel unnatural and difficult to fast for a long period of time, but the human body is well-equipped to deal with the lack of caloric intake.

Some religions and cultures incorporate fasting into their roster of practices. In the case of illness or certain medical conditions, fasting is an essential facet of healing and recovery. So let it be known that fasting is anything but dangerous, if observed properly and appropriately.

There are a lot of varieties of intermittent fasting, all using different meal schedules to either boost metabolism or increase weight loss.

The most common of all however is the 16/8 intermittent fasting schedule. Developed by Martin Berkhan, the 16/8 method is the easiest to follow and the simplest of mainstream intermittent fasting (IF) schedules.

Essentially, dieters are required to fast for around 16 hours during the day, including sleeping hours, and then restrict meals to an 8 hour window.

To put it into effect, all you really need to do is skip breakfast and push your first meal to 12 noon. From this point onwards, you can load up until 8 PM, which is the closing hour for your meal window.

Now, the clincher - should you observe a caloric restriction when observing intermittent fasting? The answer is *yes*.

Although Intermittent Fasting doesn't call for such strict limitations when it comes to your intake of food, it does put a cap on how much you can eat. After all, eating more than your body needs will result to weight gain no matter what kind of diet you're on.

Fortunately for weight watchers though, intermittent fasting simply requires individuals to stay within their normal caloric limits, in order to maintain weight loss achieved through the ketogenic diet.

What should you eat when you're observing intermittent fasting?

A lot of people who put their weight in the hands of Intermittent Fasting choose to eat virtually anything they can get their hands on.

So whether it's a fat packed cheeseburger in a homemade cauliflower bun, or a full on carb-loaded pasta dinner, the sky's the limit. The only thing you need to consider is the fact that the results might be compromised if you choose a diet that's too heavy on carbs.

The keto diet and intermittent fasting both help manage your weight by putting your system in a state of starvation.

During keto, you're starved of carbohydrates, forcing your body to look for energy elsewhere. Your body enters a state of metabolic stress called ketosis, during which it bumps up the burning of fat storage, as a means to fuel your functions.

During intermittent fasting, starvation is caused by fasting. For a large portion of the day, you won't have anything introduced into your system, so if you're only eating the bare minimum, your body will burn through it as you go throughout your day, and will be left with nothing for a large portion of the fasting period.

This pushes your body into starvation mode - much like when you're on a ketogenic diet - forcing your system to use up any fat reserves.

However, unlike keto, intermittent fasting can be slightly less stable. This is especially true if you're eating more carbs and proteins during the meal window.

Unlike keto, which requires that you eat mostly fat to keep your body in a constant state of ketosis, intermittent fasting doesn't aim to keep you constantly in starvation mode. That is, your body will only burn up fat stores several hours after your last meal for your available window.

So what does that mean?

If you eat *more carbs and proteins* for your meals, your body might have more than enough to work with throughout the day - even during your fasting phase. So starvation will only really occur after around 12 hours have passed from the last time you ate.

If you're following the 16/8 method, then that only leaves you around 4 hours left to tap into your fat reserves, before you eat your next meal. From the standpoint of weight loss, it doesn't look like such a promising technique.

The purpose of intermittent fasting in this case isn't to help you lose more weight, but to help you keep off the weight you lost with keto.

While there are a lot of individuals who have successfully increased their weight loss results by combining both keto and intermittent fasting, it's important to remember that you need to give your body a break from the fat-intensive meals that are required under the parameters of keto. This is to simply prevent the potential risks that come with long-term carbohydrate starvation.

To help make the most of your intermittent fasting eating schedule, consider planning well-balanced healthy meals that incorporate mostly proteins and fiber.

Protein is known to keep individuals feeling fuller for longer after each meal, and fiber does the same. This should make the fasting phase a lot easier to stick to, especially during the first few weeks.

If you're wondering whether you should incorporate any carbohydrates into your new diet schedule, consider this - carbohydrates can increase the strength and frequency of hunger pangs and cravings.

If you remember some of the information shared in earlier chapters, one of the main issues of consuming carbs is the inevitable sugar crash. Eating too much carbs during your meal window means that you might fall victim to painful hunger pangs and aggressive cravings later on in the day during the fasting phase of your diet. This makes it more difficult to maintain the fast, pushing dieters to grab unwarranted meals, even when they're supposedly out of their meal window.

Experts recommend keeping carbohydrates to a maximum of 30% of your meals, with proteins and fibers taking up most of the portions. You can also add in some fat, if you prefer, but it's always encouraged that you choose whole foods that have the highest possible nutritional value, to manage your health.

If carbs are so difficult to manage, why should they be a part of the diet in the first place?

The answer is simple - our bodies need carbohydrates.

The simple fact that you're shifting from keto to a new dietary plan means that you acknowledge the danger of staying on keto for too long.

Our bodies were designed to use all of the other macronutrients and micronutrients available - not just those found in fats. So, providing it what it needs, even in small amounts, will help prevent the chances of malnutrition or nutritional deficiencies as time wears on.

Other Intermittent Fasting Schedules

If you're eating a diet that's mainly made up of carbs and proteins, you might find that intermittent fasting's effects will only occur a few hours towards the end of your fasting window.

This is likely because the amount of food you eat during the meal window is sufficient to see you through an extended period of time, overlapping with your supposed fasting period.

While that should be enough to help maintain your weight, there are some people who might still gain a few extra pounds, despite following through with the 16/8 intermittent fasting schedule.

The reason may be one of the following:

Eating too much

If you consume more food than your body needs, it's possible to store more of it than you burn during the fasting period. Even though you might be observing the diet schedule strictly, eating more than you actually use will force your system to store the excess, defeating the purpose of your new dietary plan.

Your fasting window isn't long enough

The reason why the fasting window is typically longer than the meal window, is so that your body is given enough time to enter a semi-starvation state to encourage it to tap into other energy reserves.

108

Because everyone is different, it could take some people faster or longer to achieve this. For instance, more active dieters might find themselves burning fat just a few hours into their fasting period, while those who have a more sedentary lifestyle might only start burning fat a few hours before the fasting period ends.

Lengthening the fast can make it more likely to burn extra fat, and reduce the amount of food you're allowed to consume, since you'd consequently have a shorter meal phase.

Choosing the wrong foods

Although it is true that the intermittent fasting diet doesn't call for any specific food choices, selecting healthy foods should be a no-brainer. Whole, natural, organic food choices are recommended for proper bodily functioning and optimum wellness.

There are some people who think that the loose parameters set by the intermittent fasting diet mean they can eat anything at any amount, but that isn't essentially true.

The diet maintains that you need to eat healthy, whole food choices and keep junk food to a minimum. This way, you can get the best results out of your effort and prevent weight gain.

If you find that the 16/8 schedule is causing problems with the results you want to achieve, you can try a different intermittent fasting schedule and find out which one your body adjusts to the best.

Let's take a look at some other fasting schedules.

The 5:2 Diet

One of the more popular alternatives to the 16/8 IF schedules is the 5:2 diet. The plan entails eating normally for 5 days of the week, and then restricting your intake to just 500-600 calories two days every week.

The principle behind the schedule is that you're unlikely to gain weight if you're not eating more than you should.

During the 5 days of normal dietary consumption, it's recommended that you eat just a few hundred calories below the recommended intake.

On days of fasting, women should take a total of 500 calories, while men take 600. The total number of calories on fasting days can be divided into 2 or 3 meals, depending on your preference.

These two days of extremely reduced food intake should be enough to keep your weight in check and offset any excess that you might have consumed during the five regular meal days.

What many dieters prefer about the 5:2 diet is that it isn't demanding on most days. However, a glaring downside is the sheer willpower needed to make sure you get through the 2 fasting days, without exceeding caloric restrictions.

Eating a standard diet for several days during the week and then shifting suddenly to a dramatically limited intake over 2 days can be exceptionally difficult, especially if you've been eating enough carbs during the week to cause significant hunger and cravings.

Eat-Stop-Eat

Popularized by Brad Pilon, the eat-stop-eat intermittent fasting schedule is probably the second most popular, right next to 16/8.

Unlike the previously mentioned methods, this specific routine calls for a whole 24 hour fast once or twice a week. Food consumption during the rest of the *normal* days should remain unchanged.

That is, aside from making sure you fall within the right number of calories for your weight and activity level, you're free to eat whatever you want, whenever you want. Of course, it pays to indulge in healthy food though.

To enact the eat-stop-eat method, you need to complete a 24-hour period with zero solid food intake. Coffee, tea, and other low calorie or no calorie drinks are allowed, however.

You also get to choose *when* to start your fast. Most individuals prefer fasting from dinner one day to dinner the next day. But fasting from breakfast to breakfast or lunch to lunch produces the same results.

Choosing how many times in a week you should "stop" depends on your specific preference and your own metabolic rate.

If you feel that you might have a slower metabolism compared to most other people, you might benefit from two fasting days in a week. The strategy works best when the fasts are scheduled 3 to 4 days apart, to prevent any adverse reactions.

Perhaps the main issue with the eat-stop-eat diet is that it's really not that easy to enact. The first half of the day can fly by with little trouble, but once those hunger pangs and cravings start to kick in, it can be very difficult to stick to the 24 hour fast.

Experts recommend cutting back on carbohydrates 3 meals before the beginning of the fasting period. This should help reduce cravings and appetite, and might make it easier to finish the fast, without falling off the bandwagon.

For those who might have a particularly hard time fasting the whole day without sneaking in a bite or two, it is possible to gradually work yourself into the schedule instead of trying to dive in straight away.

Working on a 16 hour fast first, and then adding hours until you complete a whole 24-hour cycle can be much easier on the body, giving you time to adjust instead of forcing you into a new routine that's drastically different from your typical practice.

The Convenience Schedule

Sometimes, it can be difficult to follow through a specific meal schedule, especially because work and personal life don't really bend to accommodate any dietary changes you might make.

So some experts recommend just fasting when convenient. Skipping a meal or two, especially if you don't feel hungry, is a great way to encourage your body to burn fat stores and an easy solution to prevent yourself from a calorie binge.

By skipping one or two meals whenever convenient, there's zero commitment to sticking to a routine, and thus no disappointment when you fail to see it through.

The problem with the convenience schedule is that there is no permanence and discipline. So, some people who might not have such a firm resolve to maintain their weight might find that they won't skip any meals at all.

The convenience schedule really works best for people who know they might have the opportunity to skip meals without having to exert too much effort into doing it.

For instance, office workers who already skip meals at their desk, or stay-at-home moms that tend to an empty home at lunchtime while the kids are in school, might have better success with the convenience schedule than most others.

Alternate Fasting

The alternate fasting schedule works as the name suggests - individuals alternate between fasting days and regular days.

Every other day, dieters are urged to eat the bare minimum which is around 500 calories for women and 600 for men. The day after fasting, they can revert back to their standard diet.

While it has been found to be an effective weight management solution, fasting every other day can be a big challenge for most people. So this advanced technique might be better reserved for those who have the kind of willpower and determination needed to stick to a diet that's exceedingly restrictive.

On top of being a challenge for daily observance, the alternate fasting schedule might also pose a few issues in terms of long-term sustainability.

Going to bed several nights in a week with a gurgling tummy might not seem like a feasible long-term situation for most folks.

The Warrior Diet

Patterned after the dietary practices of warriors from ancient times, the warrior diet entails eating very little in the morning and then feasting over a 4-hour window in the evening.

This daily fast looks a lot like the 16/8 schedule, with the main distinction being that it doesn't have such a large window of opportunity for eating.

During the day, dieters are encouraged to consume small servings of fresh fruits, vegetables, and low calorie or zero calorie beverages like coffee, tea, and water. In the evening, a 4-hour meal window is allowed, allowing individuals to consume as much as they can during the time frame.

Another thing that sets the warrior diet apart from other intermittent fasting schemes is that it does impose one other restriction, and that involves food choices.

For other schedules, *any* food can be a suitable inclusion as long as it's healthy and whole. For the warrior diet, individuals are encouraged to eat food similar to what they would consume on a paleo diet.

Choices that resemble their natural condition prior to being processed and packed for human consumption are highly recommended, to achieve the best results with this specific strategy.

Sure, there are lots of other intermittent fasting schedules out there. But choosing the best one ultimately depends on your own body's response to the strategy and on your strength of willpower.

Sticking to an intermittent fasting schedule can feel clumsy and prone to errors at the start, especially if you're coming from a ketogenic diet that let you eat anything and everything you wanted.

To avoid failure and disappointment, avoid incorporating changes too drastically.

Slow and steady is often much more sustainable, making it easier for you to keep going, as you gradually turn up the intensity over time.

9

MAINTAINING YOUR WEIGHT

One of the best ways to keep your weight in constant check is to alternate between intermittent fasting and the ketogenic diet.

The former helps maintain your weight during normal seasons of your life, while the latter helps you blast off fat that you might have gained during certain periods of increased food intake.

So when should you be on keto and when should you be intermittent fasting?

The answer is simple - go ketogenic if you're preparing for a major event like a wedding, or if you're getting geared up for bikini season. Keto also works as a great way to burn away fat that might have been gained over a short period of time, like a birthday week, Thanksgiving, or Christmas.

Any other time of the year, you might want to adapt an intermittent fasting schedule. This should help maintain your weight and prevent you from gaining any extra weight.

In case you do pack on a few extra pounds during the normal seasons in your life though, you can always rotate the ketogenic diet to help burn away what was gained.

There are some instances however when the switch between intermittent fasting and the ketogenic diet might seem a little confusing. Consider this example:

A woman weighed herself and realized that she had gained 36 pounds in the past year. Now she's hoping to utilize the keto diet to her benefit and lose the weight she gained to re-establish her previously slimmer physique.

Question: Given that she might only lose a maximum of 23 pounds after 21 days of observing the keto diet, should she try to extend the journey to shave off the 36 pounds completely?

The short answer is *no*. In any case, dieters are discouraged from observing keto for more than 3 months given the dangers that it might pose.

In fact, even the original developer of the diet administered it to his patients in cycles, giving them breaks of normal dietary practices in between each cycle. This gives the body time to adjust and assume normal functioning, taking it out of starvation mode, to avoid any long-term problems.

If the woman in our example wants to lose 36 pounds, she can start off with the 21-day ketogenic diet and then switch to intermittent fasting, applying a more aggressive deficit in her caloric intake to help her shave off what's left of her original 36 pound excess.

Remember, although the intermittent fasting method is typically used for weight maintenance, it's a highly adaptable strategy. That said, it can be used for weight loss as long as you edit the numbers just right.

Another issue that some dieters might encounter is the time frame it takes to fully recover from a fat-intensive diet.

That is, how soon can you get back on keto after adapting an intermittent fasting schedule? Consider this example:

After having completed the 21-day keto diet, Jonah managed to get rid of the extra pounds he gained over the holidays and New Year's. He started in late January and ended his diet towards the end of February.

But with spring break approaching, he wants to get back to keto after just two weeks of intermittent fasting, so he can show off a flab-free body at the beach.

Question: Is it too soon to restart keto knowing that he's only been off of the diet for 2 weeks?

The answer is *yes*, it's too soon. It takes your body around 3 weeks to become accustomed to a new diet.

That's why the keto diet works so well at the 3 week mark - because that's just around the time that your body becomes fully adapted to the change. Extending keto beyond that could limit the fat loss you experience, since your body would have become too accustomed.

In the same way, you should wait at least 3 weeks before you restart the keto diet from your intermittent fasting strategy.

This helps make sure that you've completely recovered from the changes that keto caused on your system, so you can avoid the long-term effects that ketosis might have on your body.

Then, of course, there's the question of whether it's important to revert back to the ketogenic diet or if it's possible to only complete one cycle.

Take this scenario for example:

The last time Margot tried the ketogenic diet was a year and a half ago. After the diet, she lost 19 pounds and has since adopted a 16/8 intermittent fasting diet.

Her weight has remained generally the same throughout all that time, even after all the holidays, birthdays, and parties she's attended.

Question: Should she revert back to the keto diet on a routine schedule (after the holidays, before summer)?

The answer is *no*. If there's no need to blast fat, then there's no need for keto.

Although it is an exceptionally effective weight loss strategy, you don't really need to observe keto, if you don't need to lose weight.

Many of the other benefits of the diet can be achieved through less drastic means, so if you were hoping to attain all of the other advantages aside from weight loss, there are easier alternatives.

If intermittent fasting has proven to be an effective weight management or weight loss strategy for you, then perhaps there's no need to make any changes to your current dietary techniques. As long as you're eating healthy and you're feeling well, then you're doing just fine.

That said, it's important to ask yourself at the beginning of any diet - "Do I really need to lose weight?" Often times, people romanticize the idea of weight loss, often thinking it's the healthy option. But not all weight loss is healthy.

If you've been able to maintain yourself at a healthy weight for years, if you feel generally well, and if you don't see any issues with the way you look, then there might not be a need to lose weight in the first place.

More often than not, we give in to the external pressure, because weight loss is seen as a prize to some, even if it is not always needed. Assess your own situation before starting on weight loss to make sure that you're not forcing your body into an impossible condition.

While keto and intermittent fasting are generally safe as long as you follow the guidelines and parameters of each diet, they may become unsafe if weight loss was unnecessary in the first place.

That said, if you or someone you know is struggling with issues concerning body image, make sure to direct them to a counselor or a support group that can help them address the issue.

Not all weight loss is healthy - avoid falling victim to criticism that might distort your personal idea of your own health and wellness.

LISA SCOTT

10

WHY WAIT?

From aggressive weight loss, to improved clarity of thought, to enhanced cardiovascular health, and many other things in between, the ketogenic diet provides a number of impressive benefits that make it more than just another fad diet.

Proving throughout the years that it is here to stay, keto has cemented its place in the ever changing and advancing realm of weight loss.

So, in the face of revolutionary fat burning supplements, enticing fad diets, and even weight loss surgery, the ketogenic diet remains a garrison for those who want real results over a short period of time.

Of course, it's not without its downsides. But don't all diets pose risks?

Making sure that you observe the ketogenic diet for no more than 21 days can help curb the long-term dangers and keep you healthy and safe without having to give up the promising outcomes that the strategy provides.

With hundreds of thousands that vouch for keto, and millions more on their way to reaping their ketogenic diet harvest, there's no better time to get your weight loss journey started.

Just make sure to use the information in this book as a guide. Always consult with your physician before you adopt any major changes in your diet - ketogenic or otherwise.

Are you ready for that whole body transformation? Do you want to finally walk with confidence?

If you're ready to reimagine yourself and bring out the best of your health and physique, then the time is now.

Why wait? Make that first step today to transform yourself - you won't regret it!

11

FRENCH-INSPIRED KETO RECIPES - INCLUDING SLOW COOKER AND CROCKPOT RECIPES

One of the best ways to make living the Keto lifestyle easy, is to plan to eat some delicious foods.

Cooking in a slow cooker or crockpot is one way to bring out some amazing flavors in your food. Cooking this way can also be a great time saver, as you can just throw the ingredients in together and come back hours later, and find a delicious meal, ready to eat!

Tips For Adapting Any Recipe for your Slow Cooker or Crockpot

Here's some tips for adapting any stew or casserole recipe for your crockpot:

- brown the meat, before adding to the pot

- your slow cooker should be between 1/2 full and 2/3 full

- ensure that meat and vegetables are covered with stock or liquid

- as the stock won't evaporate, you may need to add a thickening during the cooking process (for example, flour) or at the end of the cooking process (for example, cream)

- for each hour you'd cook the recipe in the oven or on the hob, allow 8 hours on low or 4 hours on high

- if you need to add ingredients towards the end of cooking, add about 30 minutes before you want to eat

- don't lift the lid if you don't need to - this loses heat and prolongs the cooking time

French-Inspired Keto Recipes

If any country knows how to cook, it's the French. They are big on flavor and are a well-known for being a nation of food-lovers.

Julia Child brought the wonders of French cooking to the American nation, with her book 'Mastering the Art of French Cooking' and we've been fascinated with their fabulous dishes ever since.

So, to get you started on your keto journey, what better than some tasty recipes, inspired by some French classic recipes and favorite dishes?

Here's some of my favourite recipes, that I hope you'll enjoy cooking, to create bistro cooking in your own home.

Each of the following recipes serves 4 persons, unless otherwise indicated.

Beef Stew (Boeuf Bourguignon)

Ingredients

> 1.5 tbsp oil
>
> 2 tbsp butter
>
> 125g bacon, chopped roughly
>
> 50g beef brisket or chuck roast, cut into cubes
>
> 2 carrots, chopped
>
> 1 large onion, sliced
>
> 1 garlic clove
>
> 2 tbsp flour
>
> 500 ml red wine
>
> 250 ml beef stock
>
> 1 bouquet garni
>
> 250g baby mushrooms
>
> salt and pepper

Preparation

- Fry onions and chopped bacon in the oil and melted butter. Drain and add to slow cooker.

- Add the cubed beef and flour, cooking until the beef is browned on all sides. Transfer to the slow cooker.

- Add in the carrots, garlic, mushrooms, bouquet garni, red wine and beef stock, together with seasoning.

- Cook for 6-8 hours on low

- Serve with mashed celeriac or celery root

Chicken in Wine (Coq Au Vin)

Ingredients

100g chopped bacon or lardons

1 tbsp butter

2 tbsp flour

1.5kg chicken, jointed - or 4 pieces of chicken

250ml dry white wine

100ml chicken stock

1 bay leaf

2 garlic cloves, chopped

250g shallots, chopped

2 celery stalks, sliced

1 large carrot, chopped

150g baby mushrooms

Salt and pepper

Preparation

- Fry the lardons or bacon, in the butter, until golden. Remove and add to the slow cooker.

- Fry the chicken and flour in the remaining butter, until golden on all sides.

- Remove the chicken and add to the slow cooker.

- Add the white wine, bay leaf, garlic, shallots, celery and carrot. Season with salt and pepper.

- Cover and cook on low for 6 hours.

- Before serving, fry the onions in a little butter, until golden. Serve the chicken and scatter the onions over the top of the dish.

French Omelette (serves 1)

Ingredients

> 2 large eggs
>
> 2 tbsp milk or water
>
> 40g butter
>
> freshly chopped flat-leaf parsley (optional)
>
> handful of chopped ham (optional)
>
> salt and pepper

Preparation

- Mix eggs, milk/water, salt and pepper in a bowl. Beat well.

- Melt butter in omelette pan, until very hot and sizzling

- Pour in egg mixture, using a fork to stir the eggs in a circular motion

- As the omelette starts to set, use the fork to move the cooked portions to the centre of the pan, so that the uncooked eggs cook on the hot pan

- Cook until omelette is set on the bottom, and slightly soft on the top

- Sprinkle on the filling (herbs or ham), then fold the omelette in half.

- Serve immediately

Seafood Stew (Bouillabaisse)

Ingredients

20oz canned crushed tomatoes

1/2 cup white wine

2 cups vegetable stock

3 cloves garlic, chopped

1/2 onion, sliced

1 celery stick, sliced

1/2 tsp dried thyme

1/2 tsp dried basil

1/2 tsp dried cilantro

salt and pepper

1kg seafood (for example, fish, mussels, prawns)

Preparation

- Add all the ingredients into the slow cooker, except the seafood

- Cook in the slow cooker on low for 4-6 hours

- Add the seafood and turn on to high

- Cook for 45-60 minutes, until seafood is thoroughly cooked

- Serve hot

Duck Confit (Confit de Canard)

Ingredients

4 duck legs

1/4 cup olive oil

Salt and pepper to taste

Preparation

- Arrange the duck legs in a dish and season generously with salt and pepper. Cover and refrigerate over night.
- Pour olive oil in the bottom of the slow cooker.
- Place the duck legs in a single layer, in the slow cooker. Cook on low for 6 hours.
- Transfer the duck legs and fat to a separate pan. Cover and refrigerate.
- When ready to serve, fry the legs in a pan, until warmed through, on both sides.
- Serve with low carb vegetables, such as broccoli or cauliflower.

Duck a l'orange

Ingredients

2 duck breasts

5 oranges

1 apple, peeled, cored and sliced

1 onion, sliced

salt and pepper

Preparation

- Cut the duck breasts in half. Place on the bottom of the slow cooker. Season with salt and pepper.
- Peel two of the oranges and break into sections. Add the sections to the slow cooker.
- Juice the remaining three oranges, and add to the slow cooker.
- Add the apple and onion.
- Cook on low for 6-8 hours

French Onion Pork Chops

Ingredients

1/2 tbsp butter

4 pork chops

1 onion, sliced

1 can French Onion soup

Salt and pepper

Preparation

- Fry the pork chops and onion in the butter, until chops are cooked on both sides.
- Place in the slow cooker, with seasoning.
- Add the soup.
- Add up to 1/2 cup of water, to cover the chops, if needed
- Cook on low for 4 hours.
- Serve hot!

Sole Meunière

Ingredients

> 4 filets of sole, about 100g each
>
> 80g flour
>
> salt and pepper
>
> 90g butter
>
> Juice of 3 lemons
>
> 1/2 tsp lemon zest

Preparation

- Heat the plates, ready to serve the fish.
- Dip the fillets in the flour, salt and pepper
- Over a medium heat, melt butter in a skillet or sauté pan.   Heat until it just starts to turn brown.
- Place the seasoned floured fillets in the butter. Fry for 2 minutes, before turning over.
- Add the lemon juice and zest to the pan. Cook second side for a total of 2 minutes.
- Remove fish from the skillet or pan, and pour juices from the pan over
- Serve hot!

Warm Bacon and Egg Salad (Salade Lyonnaise)

Ingredients

  1 tbsp oil

  5 slices bacon, cut into 1/2 inch strips

  225g frisee lettuce, chopped or torn into bite-size pieces

  4 eggs

Dressing

  1 shallot, chopped

  1 tbsp red wine vinegar

  1 tbsp mustard

  3 tbsp olive oil

  salt and pepper

Preparation

- Fry the bacon strips in the oil, until bacon is crispy and golden brown. Remove from pan and drain.

- Whisk the shallot, vinegar, mustard together. Pour in oil gradually, to make a thick dressing. Add salt and pepper, as required

- Poach the four eggs.

- Whilst eggs are cooking, toss the leaves and dressing together.

- Serve eggs, on bed of salad and bacon strips, drizzled with any remaining dressing

Mussels in Wine (Moules Marinières)

Ingredients

2kg mussels (prepared)

300ml dry white wine

1 onion, sliced

salt and pepper

Preparation

- Discard any mussels with open shells or broken shells
- Pour the wine and onions into a saucepan and bring to the boil. Add salt and pepper, to taste.
- Add the mussels and cover the pan. Cook for 3-4 minutes.
- Your dish is ready to serve, once all the mussels have opened. Discard any unopened mussels.
- Serve hot.

Nicoise Salad

Ingredients

4 eggs

2 cups romaine lettuce, shredded

2 x 6oz cans tuna

225g green beans

1/2 red onion, sliced

15 cherry or grape tomatoes, halved

2 tbsp oil

2 tbsp vinegar

salt and pepper

Preparation

- Hard boil the eggs and set aside to cool. Cut into quarters.

- Lightly cook the green beans, until soft.

- Mix together the oil and vinegar in a jar, together with salt and pepper. Shake well, until mixed.

- To assemble the salad, add the lettuce as the base, then top with the eggs, tuna chunks, beans and tomatoes.

- Drizzle with the oil and vinegar dressing.

- Serve

Chicken Cordon Bleu Casserole

Ingredients

1 rotisserie chicken or cooked chicken, chopped into bite-size pieces

200g smoked deli ham, chopped into bite-size pieces

200g cream cheese

1 tbsp Dijon mustard

1 tbsp white vinegar

250g shredded cheddar cheese

Preparation

- Heat oven to 400F, 200C

- In a bowl, mix the cream cheese, mustard, vinegar and most of cheese (reserving 50g of cheese for the topping). Stir in chicken and ham pieces.

- Spoon into a baking dish and top with remaining cheese.

- Bake for 10-15 minutes or until cheese is golden

- Serve with a fresh salad on the side

Chicken Fricassee

Ingredients

1 tbsp oil

2 onions, chopped

2 garlic cloves, crushed

200g celery sticks

250g chestnut mushrooms, sliced

2 lemons

400g chicken breast pieces

200ml chicken stock

150ml cream

Preparation

- Fry the celery, onion and garlic in the oil. Add chicken pieces and fry until golden on all sides.

- Add the sliced mushrooms, and cook for a further 3-4 minutes.

- Add in chicken stock and simmer for 15-20 minutes.

- Just before serving, stir in cream and warm through, then serve hot with low-carb vegetables

Salmon and Steamed Vegetables

Ingredients

1 tbsp olive oil

4 pieces of fresh salmon

Juice of 1 lemon

250g French beans, trimmed

250g courgettes, sliced

1/2 cauliflower, cut into florets

1/2 head of broccoli, cut into florets

50g butter

Salt and pepper

Preparation

- Preheat the oven to 200°C, 180°C fan, GM6.

- Brush four squares of foil, each large enough to wrap a salmon fillet, with olive oil.

- Place the fish on the foil, drizzle a little oil and lemon juice over and season with salt and pepper. Wrap foil loosely and place on a baking tray.

- Bake in oven for 12-15 minutes.

- Steam the vegetables and serve with melted butter.

Lamb Stew (Navarin d'Agneau

Ingredients

1kg shoulder of lamb, cut into large chunks

2 tbsp oil

1 onion, chopped

2 cups lamb stock (or chicken or beef stock)

1 cup white wine (optional)

Bouquet garni or bay leaf

4 carrots, sliced

1 cup butternut squash, chopped into chunks

1 cup frozen peas

salt and pepper

Preparation

- In a pan, brown the lamb pieces in the oil. Drain and add the lamb to the slow cooker.

- Fry the onion, until softened, then add to the slow cooker.

- Add in the stock, white wine, bouquet garni or bay leaf and seasoning.

- Cook for 1 hour on high
- Reduce heat to low and add in carrots, butternut squash and peas. Cook on low for a further 5 hours.

Get Cooking!

Hopefully some of the recipes above have got your tastebuds tingling and your imagination going.

I hope that you're thinking that this keto journey might not be so bad after all.

Especially, as some of the dishes (that is, beef bourgignon, lamb stew and coq au vin) have plenty of wine in them, which makes for an incredible flavor!

Throughout this book, you've learned the science behind why keto works, you've heard of some of the typical keto mistakes and you've found out how intermittent fasting can help you keep the weight off.

Your keto journey really can be fun - especially if you start off with some of these amazing recipes to enjoy. If you do, it certainly won't feel like you're depriving yourself!

So, it's time to stop reading and start cooking. It's time for you to take the next step on your keto weight loss journey!

As the French might say, 'Bonne Chance', which means good luck!

I hope that you'll have the success that you dream of, when you try the Keto diet for yourself.

12

ONE MORE THING

If you've enjoyed this book and found it useful, please consider leaving a rating or review.

Thank you!

LISA SCOTT

13

MEDITERRANEAN DIET SECRETS

Author, Lisa Scott, has also written about the Mediterranean Diet and Lifestyle.

Here's the introduction, from her book, *Mediterranean Diet Secrets,* a quick start guide to healthy, anti-inflammatory food for long-lasting weight loss, with lifestyle secrets, 70 delicious recipes, cookbook and easy 14-day Meal Plan.

Introduction

What if you could find a diet, that was easy to follow, helped you lose weight and tasted great?

What if that diet also helped you to live better, for longer?

Sounds too good to be true, right?

The Mediterranean diet is not about counting calories.   In fact, the Mediterranean diet is not really a diet at all – it's a lifestyle.

It's all about the food you eat, what physical activities you participate in, and how you socialize with family and friends.

Most restrictive diets aim to act as quick fixes. They promise to deliver results, fast.

Sometimes these diets work but, more often than not, it's just a temporary fix. You end up reverting back to the old ways, eating the wrong types of foods and gaining the weight right back again.

The Mediterranean diet is about making a real change to your life. It's about preventing disease and decay. It's a way of life, that can reduce your chance of diseases such as cancer, heart disease and diabetes.

Remember how good it feels when you go on vacation in the sunshine? It's great to eat fabulous food, relax and enjoy life. You return home feels refreshed and rested, with your body feeling vibrant and alive.

What if you could incorporate some of this feeling into your everyday life? What if you could eat delicious meals, take time to relax and regularly enjoy spending time out in nature or with family and friends?

Do you think that would make a difference to how you feel? Do you think that your body and mind would benefit from the change in your diet and lifestyle?

Of course they would!

So many diets take just one aspect of our life, such as diet or exercise, and suggest that changing a single aspect can impact your life.

The Mediterranean diet is different. It's a holistic approach, which focuses on the whole person, rather than any one aspect of your life.

The Mediterranean diet is a lifestyle, that focuses on more than just what you eat. It's about taking life one step at a time, embracing community, being more mindful and involved with what you eat.

It's a diet that can give you more life in your years, keeping you mentally and physically active for longer.

It's about a new way of living, about developing new healthier habits that can last a lifetime. It's about eating great-tasting foods that make you feel vibrant and alive.

Let's compare that, for a moment, with the traditional diets you might have tried in the past.

The Problem With Traditional Diets

Our society seems to have the idea that things are designed to be used up, thrown away, then replaced.

There's a focus on speed, on how something can be quickly achieved, with little emphasis on taking the time to enjoy life.

We all want to live a fulfilling life, we may even know what it takes, but few of us have the patience it takes to really find discipline in our lives to do what's needed.

We might choose the solution of quick diet pills, extreme exercise, or "cleanses", some of which come with unpleasant side-effects. These things can work, but only for a short time.

Most diets offer a short, sharp fix, but don't do anything to change the underlying problem, that is, your unhealthy lifestyle and diet.

The reason why so many of us find that we can't lose weight or keep the pounds off, is because we're expecting that quick fix. We're not willing to give any long-term commitment that might make a real difference to our life.

In order to live a healthier life, it's more than just about the food you eat. There needs to be a real shift in the way you go about your day-to-day life.

Most of us are living life at a breakneck speed, feeling stressed and out-of-control.

The impact of modern living has made us feel as if we can't do anything to change the way we live.

We work 9 to 5 jobs, go home and do the chores, only to have to go to sleep feeling tired and wake up early the next morning, only to do it all again.

We find ourselves trapped in an unhappy cycle. It can feel as if we just don't have the time to make any change to our lives. We certainly don't have time to follow yet another diet!

It might seem like you have to go to the gym every night, try the latest diets and buy a bunch of new cookbooks in order to see the results you want.

But there is a solution, a way of the merry-go-round of life and it's much simpler than you might imagine: it's called the Mediterranean diet.

The Mediterranean diet is easy to maintain. It can fill you with energy, helps you lose weight and is great for your health and wellbeing.

If you follow the Mediterranean diet and lifestyle, you won't have to worry about crazy side-effects from your diet. You won't have to worry about gaining back all that weight you lost.

Eating healthy foods will become a habit, something you barely even think about.

Unlike some other diets, there's nothing extreme about the Mediterranean diet. No fad dieting, no crazy exercising, just a sustainable, enjoyable life, that you'll learn to love.

All you need is a desire to change or a passion for finding a better lifestyle.

The Mediterranean diet has been proven over decades, by millions of people. It works. It's a long term solution to your health and weight issues, rather than a quick fix.

It's not something a doctor has created, but something that scientists discovered, after looking at the lives of real people.

After a few days on the Mediterranean diet, you'll start to feel much better. Your digestion will regulate, your breathing will get easier, and you'll feel much better in general.

You might not look in the mirror after a week and see a dramatic weight loss; but let's get real, is there really a diet that's actually going to do that for you long-term?

The Mediterranean diet can produce permanent weight loss, but it's not going to happen overnight. It can help you maintain your weight too, something few diets actually address.

It's a diet that's not only filling, but also tastes delicious. When it tastes this good, it makes it easy to maintain your diet. In fact, you'll probably forget you're on a diet at all.

You aren't even going to feel hungry. We've become used to the idea that dieting about feeling permanently hungry. We can feel anxious, thinking that we'll have to give up the foods we like, or feel hungry, in order to see the results we want.

The Mediterranean diet is filled with foods that are rich and filling, so you never have to worry about going hungry.

If you love to snack, this diet will be right up your street. Snacking is actually encouraged in a Mediterranean diet. You can snack on nuts, seeds, and fruits. Multiple small meals a day help keep the metabolism running, often producing a higher weight loss.

The Mediterranean diet means that you don't have to give up eating foods that taste great. Instead, your goal is to make more conscious choices and decisions for your health, not for convenience.

The Mediterranean diet doesn't feel like just a diet. It's a change of lifestyle. It's not another book to read and follow for a few weeks, it's a way of life that can help you feel more vibrant, prevent common diseases and prolong your life expectancy.

Many popular diets leave people hungry, hopeless, and disappointed. That's why they're called 'fad' diets - they come and go, because they're simply not workable and require a strict, disciplined food or exercise regime.

The Mediterranean diet is all-inclusive. Anyone can participate, and it doesn't take anything but a willingness to try new things. It's a diet that the whole family can eat - no more cooking one thing for them and another for you.

The best way to get started with a Mediterranean diet is to include family members, if you can. With your family on board with your healthy lifestyle, it's more likely there will be a positive outcome.

Having a support system that you can depend on really comes in handy, especially when experiencing a significant change in your lifestyle.

Eating healthily with others, can help prevent you sliding back into your old ways, getting fast food and sitting in front of the television while you eat.

Like any change in your life, the Mediterranean diet may not be easy at first, it'll probably take some work to make the changes; but eventually, it will become an easy and enjoyable way of life.

The Mediterranean diet is something that you can live on for life, without ever having to feel deprived. For those people living around the Mediterranean, it's their way of life.

Please note, I am not a professional nutritionist or someone with a medical degree. Any changes you make to your life, you are responsible for. When going through any significant diet and lifestyle changes, it is always best to consult a physician to ensure there won't be any health risks.

Although the Mediterranean diet is low-risk, it's still best to seek professional medical care to ensure this is the right diet for you.

I know, from personal experience, that following the Mediterranean diet can drastically help a person lose weight, maintain that weight loss, and be a much happier person overall. That's what's so great about the Mediterranean diet.

Whether you are vegan, vegetarian, or pescatarian, or have other dietary restrictions, the Mediterranean diet can work for you.

Don't worry, if the thought of eating olives or hummus scares you off, there are plenty of other foods you can enjoy!

Once you've read this book, you'll be ready to embark on your journey towards a healthy Mediterranean life.

Over the next few chapters you'll:

- have a comprehensive understanding of what the Mediterranean diet is

- understand some of the science and health benefits behind it

- know what foods can be eaten and which foods to cut down on or avoid

- be able to check out quick-start 14-day meal plan, complete with recipes

- discover how to embrace the Mediterranean diet and lifestyle for life

If you're up for the challenge of living a new, healthier way that will give you energy, help you stay healthy and lose weight, download her book now.

70216140R00089

Made in the USA
Columbia, SC
20 August 2019